INTRODUCT

THE UNPARALLEL LIVES OF THR

JOHN KEATS (17?
HENRY STEPHENS (1796-1864) and
GEORGE WILSON MACKERETH (1793-1869)

PENCRAFT, POETRY and PERSISTENT PRACTICE

by
W.S. PIERPOINT

Three of the medical apprentices who presented themselves for enrolment at the United Teaching Hospitals of Guy's and St Thomas' (Southwark, London) in October, 1815, were thrown together in digs, by chance. Friendships of different degrees were established, as their interests and careers developed in different directions. Their lives ran in unparallel courses, but intertwined closely at least for the 12 months or so that their medical instruction, leading to qualification as apothecaries and surgeons, lasted. This interaction is always described when the tragically short life of John Keats, who quickly abandoned medical practice for poetry, is described.

In his old age Henry Stephens left a brief memoir on Keats which is a major source of information on the poet's adolescent life; by that time he too had witnessed misfortune and had abandoned medicine in favour of a successful career as an inventor and manufacturer of inks and wood-stains. Written accounts of his life are brief and incomplete in many respects.

After qualification, the third student, George Wilson Mackereth, practised medicine all his working life in Hull and especially in the remote villages of Holderness to the east of Hull. He maintained a lifelong contact and friendship with Stephens. His daughter, Agnes, made a very successful marriage to Stephens' eldest son, Henry Charles, in 1863, producing children who developed the Stephens ink business internationally. Mackereth is mentioned in lists of Yorkshire medical men and only parenthetically in biographical accounts of Keats and Stephens. Here fuller details of his life and friendships are presented.

i

Printed in 11pt. Helvetica

J G Bryson Printer
158-162 High Road
East Finchley
London N2 9AS
www.jgbrysonprinter.co.uk

Cover illustrations

OPERATING THEATRE, St Thomas' Hospital
(Old Operating Theatre, London)

JOHN KEATS, A MINIATURE BY JOSEPH SEVERN, 1819.
(Keats House, Hampstead, London) top

HENRY STEPHENS
(The Stephens Collection) bottom left

GEORGE WILSON MACKERETH
Pencil drawing allegedly by Keats' friend Joseph Severn.
Houghton Library, Harvard University; MS Keats 10 (27) bottom right

Guy's and St Thomas' Hospitals:
How to get there

" There's my lodgings," said Mr Bob Sawyer[*], producing a card. "Lant Street, Borough; it's near Guy's, and handy for me you know."
....
" I shall find it," said Mr Pickwick[*].
" Come on Thursday fortnight, and bring the other chaps with you," said Mr Bob Sawyer, "I'm going to have a few medical fellows that night."

The Pickwick Papers, Chapter 30
Charles Dickens (1836-7)

[*] *Bob Sawyer, a medical student*
[*] *Samuel Pickwick, Founder of the Pickwick Club*

We gratefully acknowledge financial help
in the form of a grant from Guy's & St Thomas' Charity
which has enabled this book to be published.

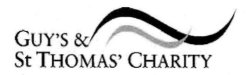

GUY'S &
St THOMAS' CHARITY

Contents

Introduction   i

Publisher's information   ii

Guy's and St Thomas'   iii

Contents   iv

List of illustrations   v

Henry Stephens   page 1

   References   28-30

John Keats   31

   References   46

George Wilson Mackereth   47

   References   58

Envoy   59

Acknowledgements   60

Index   61-62

List of Illustrations

Old Operating Theatre, London   Cover
John Keats
Henry Stephens
George Wilson Mackereth

1   Henry Stephens in later life   page 1
2   Guy's Hospital   2
3   Extract from *Endymion*   7
4   Stephens' Sonnet   8
5   Title page of Stephens' "Hernia Treatise"   14
6   Hannah Stephens' gravestone   16
7   Cholera poster   18
8   Recipe for 17c. ink   20
9   Grove House, Finchley   24
10   Farringdon Road station 1866   27
11   John Keats   31
12   St Boltoph's Without, Bishopsgate   32
13   Charles Cowden Clarke   34
14   Southwark 1815   35
15   Leigh Hunt   37
16   Keats House, Hampstead   42
17   Fanny Brawne   43
18   George Wilson Mackereth in later life   47
19   Map of the Yorkshire coastline   48
20   Owthorne Church 1806   49
21   Blue Plaque, Southwark   50
22   The Resurrection Men   51
23   Apothecaries Hall   52
24   Keyingham Church c1830   53
25   Marriage Certificate 1863   54
26   Margaret Agnes Stephens   55
27   Avenue House, Finchley   56
28   Sketch of George Wilson Mackereth   57

HENRY STEPHENS (1796-1864)

PENMANSHIP

Background and Apprenticeship

Henry Stephens was born in Holborn, London, in 1796, the second son of Joseph (1771-1820) and Catherine Stephens (1763-1843) but along with his brother John was soon moved into more rural Hertfordshire. They lived briefly in Hatfield, where sisters Frances (1798-1860) and Catherine (ca.1800) were born. Just after the turn of the century they moved to Redbourn(e), a village about five miles north of St Albans where another child, Samuel Josiah (1804–1865), was added to the family. The parents took over the running of *The Bull*, the very busy principal inn and posting-house in Redbourn High Street. The High Street sits astride Roman Watling Street and was then a major coaching route between London and the northwest. More than a hundred

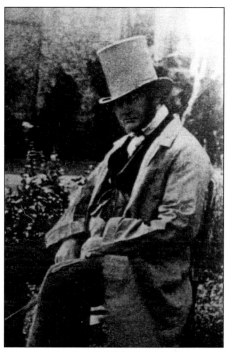

(fig 1) HENRY STEPHENS in later life about 1855

stagecoaches rattled along it day and night, many stopping to change horses and feed and refresh weary travellers[1] . It is not known how Stephens lived and was educated in this bustling and exciting environment: it may explain his love of horses and horsemanship but not his expressed wish to become a doctor.

At that time Redbourn was poorly served by doctors, and the local vestry only appointed a paid doctor for the poor in 1812[2]. In 1810 or 1811 Stephens was therefore apprenticed to an established practice in nearby Markyate about three miles north of Redbourn and on the border with Bedfordshire. He was under the instructions of John Winkfield (surgeon) and Benjamin Somers (apothecary). He and another apprentice lodged with Winkfield who had a reputation as a "wit and social character".[1] He seems to have been happy there and not above playing such tricks as hiding Mrs Winkfield's best wig. Although it is not certain where the doctor lived, it was likely to have been one of two substantial Georgian houses in the High Street[3].

The duties of Stephens as an apprentice would initially have been little more than accompanying Winkfield on his rounds and helping with dressings. At the end of his 5-year apprenticeship however he would have been expected, like Keats, to have some theoretical background and be capable, for instance of diagnosing, dressing wounds and delivering babies. But before he could set himself up in practice the law now required an approved training course of lectures, six months' experience on the wards of an approved "Public Hospital, Infirmary, or Dispensary" and his satisfying the examiners of the Society of Apothecaries (LSA) as well as those of the Royal College of Surgeons (MRCS). The time and cost of the medical qualifications was not inconsiderable; it is estimated that about £1500 was spent on the medical training of John Keats[4].

Medical Studies in London
Suitably financed, Stephens exchanged his rural surroundings for the dirty, crowded streets of Southwark just across the Thames from the city of London. He enrolled as a pupil in the united teaching school of Guy's and St Thomas' Hospitals by paying his initial "Office Fee" of £1-2-0 on 14 October 1815. The two hospitals were adjacent to each other in St Thomas Street. Guy's, a relatively modern institution had

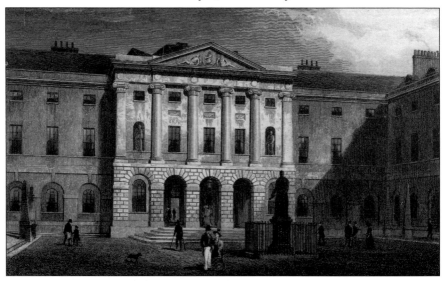

(fig 2) COURTYARD OF GUY'S HOSPITAL 1832
With statue of Thomas Guy; Engraving from a drawing by Thomas Higham

been built (1725) to remedy the overcrowding and inadequacies of the older, venerable St Thomas' (1553). But by 1815 both were crowded and their staff over-worked as, located in a crowded, unimproved and dirty area, they strove to cope with the increasing demands of the rapidly growing and industrialising city. Nevertheless there were able, energetic and liberally-minded administrators who had turned the United Hospitals into "...a magnet for the most enterprising medical practitioners of the day, and a focus for recent developments in medicine" [5]: not only were they at the cutting edge of medical research, they were helping to revolutionise social attitudes to sickness and health care. Although Stephens must have been dismayed by his translation from a quiet village to city slums, he must have been excited by the reputation and stimulation of his new environment.

He obtained convenient lodgings at 28 St Thomas Street at a house close to the hospital gates. The landlord, Markham, was a tallow-chandler, who let at least six of his upper rooms as study bedrooms and two as communal sitting rooms. Annual rent could cost up to £63 or less if sitting rooms were shared [4]. Stephens shared a sitting room with George Wilson Mackereth, a fellow student who had served his apprenticeship in Winterton, Lincs. and registered at the hospital on 4 October. On another floor, two more senior students, George Cooper and John Tyrrell, shared a sitting room with Keats. But about Christmas time both Cooper and Tyrrell left London to set up their own practices, Cooper's in Brentford. In order to save expense Keats asked Stephens and Mackereth if he could share their sitting room [4]. They readily agreed, and this arrangement seems to have lasted until November 1816, when Keats, after a holiday with his brother Tom in Margate, left to live briefly by himself in nearby Dean Street. The houses in St Thomas Street have long since been replaced but a blue plaque commemorates Keats, Stephens and the site of number 28 (fig 21).

Two days after his registration, Stephens paid the Hospital 18 guineas, the fee required to attend its wards for six months. But he had underestimated the time required to qualify for both LSA and MRCS, and had to extend his time to twelve months by paying a further six guineas on November 16. Neither Keats nor Mackereth made this mistake. Extra fees were required to attend the obligatory courses of lectures and instruction. These were delivered in two terms, lasting from October to mid-January and January 20 till mid-May annually with a short break at Christmas and a longer summer break when the weather would be too hot for anatomy and dissection. The main lecture courses included Anatomy and Physiology, the Theory and Practice of Medicine, Chemistry and Materia Medica.

Authoritative biographies of John Keats [4,5], as well as the near-contemporary memoirs of the student John Flint South [6], give detailed accounts of the lectures, the lecturers, their fees and lecture timetables. These accounts would, of course, have described the situations and activities of Stephens and Mackereth. The two distinguished lecturers that were most likely to have made a lasting impression on Stephens were Astley Cooper, senior lecturer in Anatomy, and Alexander Marcet FRS, lecturer in Chemistry [7].

Each lecture course involved about three lectures a week, leading to a very full and busy schedule. The day began at 7.30 am with lectures followed by attendance at the hospital wards, alternating daily between Guy's and St Thomas'. In the afternoon there were anatomy lectures followed by an hour of more practical dissecting. Most evenings also involved at least an hour lecture. The courses were, by the standards of the time, thorough and demanding. They were also delivered in crowded, noisy conditions. Surgical demonstrations seem especially appalling. Thus pupils were *"...packed...like herrings in a barrel"* to watch surgery being performed in St Thomas' small, steeply rising, sawdust-covered operating amphitheatre; such crowded conditions were probably stressful enough, but the discomfort of the students was nothing when compared to that of the patients who were operated on without benefit of anaesthetics and antiseptics. Even accustomed observers could be overcome [4,6].

In spite of the distressing nature of their studies in the wards and the theatre, there seems to have been a good, friendly spirit among the pupils. Keats clearly took to it and we can only assume that Stephens and Mackereth did so too. Senior pupils and "dressers", the more experienced personal assistants to the surgeons, were very helpful to the younger pupils. There was also spare time when friendships developed and were enriched in, for instance, the sitting rooms of pupils' lodgings. At such times Keats must have introduced, and dominated, conversations on poetry and poets, and the pressing political and religious and philosophical topics of the day debated. Besides, there were the more natural aspects of city life to be explored. On Thursday 9 November, for instance, they were given a day off to watch the Lord Mayor's procession on the Thames [6]. Keats, a Londoner, took the opportunity to visit his friend Cowden Clarke in Enfield where they read poetry recently received from Leigh Hunt, the radical man of letters who was to play a major role in encouraging Keats' poetic talents.

We can guess that the country boys, Stephens and Mackereth, took the opportunity to watch the extravagant pageant. On more normal occasions there were other local attractions, including bear-baiting, and just around the corner was the *King's Head,* a medieval coaching inn where the clatter of horses in the yard might have pleasantly reminded Stephens of home. Moreover, they did not need to travel far to escape the city, and in early summer 1816, while revising for exams, they relaxed and bathed in water meadows beside the New River just north of the Thames.

The presence of the hospitals encouraged some unexpected trades which added to the local, often gruesome "colour" of the neighbourhood. Thus the constant demand for anatomical specimens had encouraged local teams of body-snatchers and grave-robbers. The students seem to have been acquainted with the team of "resurrectionists" [6] led by the hoarse-voiced, drunken Bill Crouch and his brother Jack, images of whom seem to have lodged in Keats' imagination. Their trade also suggests that the presence of Markham's chandlery so close to the hospitals was more than a coincidence. One day in the warm, muggy summer of 1816 when Stephens was probably revising for his LSA examination, Bill Crouch and his colleagues deposited a corpse in 28 St Thomas Street. It was ordered by George Cooper who had left the lodgings after Christmas and who wanted to keep up his anatomical studies in Brentford. The lodgers, possibly including Stephens and Mackereth, helped Markham wax the body and place it in a hamper for delivery to Brentford by water ferry. However competent their procedure, it seems not to have enabled the corpse to hide its presence from the other passengers on the ferry [4].

On 25 July Keats had been examined and accepted as an LSA. It was expected that he would now take his exam in surgery (MRCS) to become fully qualified. However his intensely held belief in the power and value of poetry, and his developing talent were drawing him in another direction. The powerful encouragement of Leigh Hunt and his literary circle had convinced him that he should devote his life to poetry. Mackereth was examined for LSA on the same day as Keats but was rejected. Keats' success produced some sour-grapes among his fellow lodgers, and it was attributed to his knowledge of Latin which was essential in translating the Pharmacopoeia. Stephens was not confident of his own Latin and had postponed his examination to August. He was examined on the 22nd by Mr Wills and was rejected. He was probably right about his Latin but in his chagrin belittled the examination, asserting that it was not a real test of medical knowledge [4].

The blow was presumably tempered by Mackereth having failed the test and, happily, both setbacks were temporary. But it was not until the 1st of May the next year, 1817, that both men resat the exam and were approved. Whatever the standard of their Latin, their surgery was not deficient, for both were examined by the Royal College of Surgeons, in February and March 1817, and accepted as MRCS. Stephens collected his leaving certificate from Guy's around this time. It is possible that he had finished his hospital studies completely by the time he resat his LSA and had returned to London briefly for this event.

Mackereth presumably left London after May to practise in and around Hull in Yorkshire. He must have kept in close contact with Stephens. He certainly came to visit him in London about fifteen years later, but there must have been more frequent visits for their two families would be united in 1863 by the marriage of Stephens' son, Henry Charles, to Mackereth's daughter. But by July 1816 Keats, in spite of still being a surgical dresser, had gone to live with his brothers in the city, first in Poultry and then in the nearby 76, Cheapside. He had poems published in Leigh Hunt's *Examiner* and had written *On First Looking into Chapman's Homer.* His links with hospitals were all but broken and he had established firmer links with poetry and immortality.

Before this period ended, Keats and Stephens met on an occasion that Stephens later recalled (*The Asclepiad*) [8] and has often been retold with elaborations. It happened, according to Colvin [9], while Keats lived in Cheapside and Stephens was staying in London to re-sit his LSA. Stephens came over from St Thomas Street to visit Keats and they fell into familiar habits, Keats curled up in a window seat with a notebook and Stephens at his medical texts. After some scribbling Keats asked Stephens' opinion of the line
"A thing of beauty is a constant joy"
Stephens thought that *"it has the true ring, but is wanting in some way."* Keats revised and reworked the line to
"A thing of beauty is a joy forever."
and again asked: *"What think you of that, Stephens?"*
Stephens' reply, as he recounted it, was prophetic:
"That it will live forever."
Critical commentators feel that the conversation, probably relating to a real event, has been "dressed up for effect". Less critical commentators, following Martha Walsh [1] have exaggerated Stephens' contribution to the line. This seems unlikely. This opening line to *Endymion*, Keats' first epic, has the stamp of his own authority, and seems the forerunner of his mature, philosophical belief in the powers of "beauty" and poetry[5].

A thing of beauty is a joy forever:
Its loveliness increases; it will never
Pass into nothingness; but still will keep
A bower quiet for us, and a sleep
Full of sweet dreams, and health, and quiet breathing.

Endymion book 1

(fig 3) Extract from "ENDYMION" by John Keats

Stephens' friendship with Keats

Stephens and Keats shared digs for about a year from October 1815. They met occasionally after this period as when Stephens visited Cheapside and when Keats visited Redbourn in 1818, and possibly earlier [10], thus suggesting that some lasting friendship existed between them. Stephens' recollections of Keats became of great interest after Keats' tragically early death in February 1821 and when, posthumously, his genius was very slowly becoming recognised. Stephens reminisced about his friend with two men who were later to contribute to the swelling literature about Keats.

In 1847 he wrote some notes at the request of George Felton Mathew, a former friend of Keats, who gave them to Richard Monkton Milnes (later Lord Houghton), who in 1848 published the first biography of Keats. These notes and accompanying letters were printed by Rollins in 1948 [10]. Some ten years later (1856) Stephens began a long series of conversations with Sir Benjamin Ward Richardson MD FRS (1828-1896), a close and distinguished doctor friend, who quoted them in an article in his journal *The Asclepiad* in April 1884 [8]. Comments attributed to Stephens, not always flattering to Keats, are often quoted in biographies of Keats. Their relevance here is that they often tell us as much about Stephens as they do about Keats.

The two students were divided rather than united by their common interest in poetry. Stephens had written a *Sonnet to the Stars* and was later to write an (unpublished) play. But he did not have the obsessional passion of Keats, who believed writing poetry and belonging to the company of the great poets was the highest form of human endeavour. Keats dismissed Stephens' poems and his poetic judgements out of hand and behaved with a vanity and arrogance on these matters that annoyed Stephens.

Stephens was especially annoyed at the uncritical adulation of Keats by his brothers George and Tom on their frequent visits to St Thomas Street. He was almost certainly suspicious of Keats' medical advancement, his rapid promotion to a dresser for instance, possibly suspecting that he had some hidden patronage, which may well have been the case. Keats' immediate success in his LSA examination provoked sour-grapes which was exacerbated by Stephens' own failure a few weeks later; he drew attention to Keats' obvious inattention in many lectures and condemned the examination as reflecting a knowledge of Latin rather than of medicine.

There may well have been other conflicts of attitudes. Keats' radicalism and his religious disbelief were being reinforced by the artistic circles in which he increasingly moved. Andrew Motion [5] suggests that Stephens, like Keats, was *a committed free-thinker and a friend of radicals*; in spite of Stephens' later friendship with Robert Owen, this is not the impression obtained either from his career, or his daughter's memoirs or from his activities as a churchwarden in Finchley. Although socially minded and generous, Stephens was a publicly-minded establishment figure rather than a radical one. This is not a role that would have appealed to Keats.

Sonnet to the Stars

Whilst on the brilliant firmament I gaze,
My mind revolves upon the mighty mass
Of measureless creation.... In wild amaze
Thought close on thought in swift succession pass.
Till reason floats upon the surface of Eternity!
What change's and how great may be in play
Whilst I this wond'rous wilderness survey!
Each falling star may be a bulky world
Crush'd into ruin, - into chaos hurled,
Each distinct meteor that I see arise
May be a planet burning in the skies.
All the bright bodies of the sky display
Creative wisdom, and to men convey
The noblest image of the Deity.

(fig 4) "SONNET TO THE STARS", by Henry Stephens

The friendship between the young men was not one of those intimate and enduring friendships that Keats was capable of inspiring among his artistic friends. Nevertheless it seems strong and genuine enough to withstand some pride and conceit on Keats' part and some suspicion and envy on Stephens'. Moreover, the reminiscences reveal the sharpness and astuteness of Stephens' powers of observation. He noticed, for instance, that the young poet was at that stage more moved by descriptive poetry than by narrative or more emotional verse. He noted the pride and affection that he had for Georgiana, the new bride of his brother George. He also noted some stress induced in Keats by their summer bathing excursions [4,5,10], perhaps an early symptom of his predisposition to lung infections. Such close and personal observations could foretell good doctoring skills.

Stephens in Redbourn, 1817-1828
After qualification, Stephens settled in Redbourn to set up a medical practice which he developed successfully for ten years. Tradition has it that he lived in a house in the High Street just opposite the *Bull Inn* and a few yards to the south; the house, much modified and now divided, still stands adjacent to "the ruins", an ancient walled pathway that runs to Redbourn common [2]. For a few years from 1820 he was employed as doctor to the poor of Redbourn at a salary of about £50. Tradition also has it that he was popular both with the villagers and with the gentry on the large estates surrounding the village. At the Gorhambury estate he was also Vet to the hounds.

The medical problems he encountered are assumed to be those typical of a rural practice, including farming accidents. He was familiar of course with hernias and he designed a supportive truss which he boasted had been tested and approved by the best judges, agricultural labourers. He was familiar with the surgical treatment for this condition as refined and advocated by Sir Astley Cooper at Guy's, but became aware of a situation in which intestinal obstruction was not accompanied by the characteristic painful abdominal swelling. Thus he attended a local female in September 1824[1] who had these symptoms for a week and was obviously failing.

Convinced that the condition was an intestinal obstruction of some sort, he proposed an operation but was opposed by both the patient and her friends. As she deteriorated he renewed his proposal vigorously and finally successfully. He then consulted two sceptical, local colleagues, possibly including Dr Winkfield, and with their aid, operated successfully. He found an adhesion between the intestine and the body wall which was, with care, broken. Some intestinal movement was quickly restored and an apurient administered a few days later, as recommended by Astley Cooper, restored it completely and ensured the recovery of the patient. Stephens noted other, similar cases that lacked the obvious external symptoms of a strangulated hernia, but which could be equally fatal if untreated.

Emboldened by his experience he started to study the relevant published literature and became convinced that these adhesions, although they had previously been observed, were not properly appreciated nor adequately looked for in the standard surgical practice. He almost certainly consulted Astley Cooper either at Guy's or in his nearby Hertfordshire residence at Gadebridge, Hemel Hempstead. He published his opinions in a treatise [11] in 1829 about the time that the highly influential Cooper, impressed by the observations of his former pupil, had advised him not to bury himself in Redbourn, a *"mere country village"*. Stephens protested that medical and surgical knowledge *"may be cultivated as well in workhouses, pauper asylums and cottages in the country as in the vicinity of the public hospitals in London"*; but he obediently took Cooper's advice and returned to Southwark.

Stephens' treatise was published by E. Cox of St Thomas Street. It reads like the work of a bold and confident young man. It contains an appendix on *"…the cause of difference in size in the male and female bladder"*. He dismisses arguments that this is connected to matters of female delicacy, and shows that the difference also exists in species of farm animals but only after the female has been pregnant. The matter is unrelated to the hernia thesis and is not presented as quantitatively and convincingly as we nowadays expect, but it demonstrates that Stephens' interests included those of a questioning biologist who made good use of his opportunities as a rural vet. In the main text he describes, with obvious satisfaction, a hernia operation that he performed on a valued pointer bitch at the nearby Gorhambury estate. Within a few months the dog was performing well her duties in the hunting field, and Stephens was rewarded by her friendship as well as that of her aristocratic owner.

We are aware of two more events that occurred before Stephens left Redbourn permanently. First, his father died in 1820 and was buried in Redbourn Churchyard. He may have been ill for some years before his death, for his wife Catherine is listed as innkeeper of the *Bull* and a maltster from 1815 until 1826 [12]. Sale notices from 1826 give an idea of the size of the inn; there was stabling for one hundred horses. Second, John Keats briefly visited Redbourn on 22 June, 1818 [9,10]. He had lunch at the *Bull Inn* accompanied by his friend

Charles Brown with whom he was about to start his exhausting walking tour in the north, and also by his brother George Keats and his new wife Georgiana who were on their way to Liverpool to emigrate to Illinois in America. Their coach, which had set off early from Cheapside in London, stopped in Redbourn to change horses and refresh travellers. After lunch Keats sent for Stephens who came to talk to them and meet Georgiana of whom Keats was very proud.

Stephens recalled this meeting to Richardson nearly 40 years later and his account is frequently quoted because of the emotional background; Keats was exceptionally close to his two brothers, and while he was reluctantly saying farewell to George, with whom he had some financial disagreement, his younger brother Tom was terminally ill with tuberculosis in Hampstead. Also, with hindsight, Keats would over-exert himself in the Hebrides so as to compromise his own fragile lungs [5]. Some nine years later, in November 1827, Stephens copied Keats by making his own, solitary, "... *Excursion into the North*". He left a 14,000-word account of this which was prepared for publication by his great-granddaughter Jennifer Stephens in 1997 [13]. It would be inappropriate to compare this journey with that which Keats had undertaken partly to prepare his mind for the task of writing *Hyperion*.

After a spell in the backwoods of Derbyshire and one or two ill-judged rambles in the dales, Stephens visited Manchester and Liverpool to inspect their impressive civic buildings and made a coach trip back through the Welsh borders to Bristol and back to London. There were occasional moments devoted to poetic matters as when the northbound coach passed Weston Underwood near Newport Pagnell where William Cowper (1731-1800) had lived for some years. Stephens suffered little of the restless, analytical introspection that had accompanied Keats' exploration of northern Britain. His visit to a former medical student friend living in Birmingham who had fallen on hard times, although kindly meant, seems somewhat self-satisfied and patronising.

Stephens back in London (about 1829-1842)
Stephens set up his practice in a house, no. 54, at the eastern end of Stamford Street in Southwark, near the southern end of Blackfriars Bridge and not far from Guy's and St Thomas' hospitals. It was a substantial house [7] at the corner of Bennet Street. But Walsh's description of it being in a "*good residential neighbourhood*" [1] neglects its industrial components [14]: a very close neighbour was the immense steam-driven printing works of Clowes [15].

The most tragic and poorly recorded episode in Stephens' life probably occurred soon after his return to London; it concerns his first marriage and the untimely death of both his wife and baby daughter. It is not known where Hannah Woodbridge came from and how she met Stephens. Her family have not been found in Redbourn Parish records. With the aid of Pallot's Marriage Index, the wedding has been traced to Trinity Church, Marylebone (Middlesex) on 7 September 1829. Henry is recorded as "... *of the parish of Christchurch in the County of Surrey ...*"; Hannah's name is given as "*Hannah Clarke Woodbridge of the District-Rectory of St Marylebone*". Surprisingly, the wedding was witnessed by Henry's younger brother, Samuel Josiah and his wife Harriot; the short parish entry gives no evidence for the presence of any parents at the wedding. Also surprisingly the same source indicates that Samuel Josiah and his wife had been married at the same church almost a year earlier (24 August 1828) and again parents had not signed the entry as witnesses.

There can be no doubt that these records relate to the relevant Stephens family; the church is only a few hundred yards from Charlotte Street where Josiah is later known to have had a house and it is probably no coincidence that Henry and Hannah's daughter bore the same forename as Josiah's wife. The details and Marylebone background of Hannah Stephens are unknown. After her marriage she must have lived with Stephens in Stamford Street. All else that is certain about Hannah is that she died in April 1832 at the age of 28, was buried in Redbourn and that her residence was given as the parish of Christchurch in Surr(e)y.

Walsh wrote that Hannah died of consumption although the Parish Register notes that there was a local cholera epidemic at that time. Her daughter Harriot Stephens died four months before her in December 1831 exactly one year old: she too is thought to have died of consumption. Harriot seems to have spent some of her brief life in Redbourn as she was baptised there in September when she was almost nine months old although her abode, given as Christchurch, Surr(e)y, suggests that she was born in London. Thus consumption shaped the life of Stephens as it did of Keats. A loose headstone in Redbourn churchyard which once marked the common grave of mother and child bears the memorial verse written by Stephens and which was quoted by Martha Walsh [1].

Against this distressing domestic background, Stephens' practice developed. An additional activity was the revision of his hernia treatise and the production of a second edition [11]. The first edition must have met with general approval but it also attracted criticism from some reviewers. The criticisms seemed to have come from two expected directions: either there was nothing original in his work or he was advocating a risky surgical operation rather recklessly. He felt both criticisms keenly and refuted his critics robustly. He produced a new, defensive preface for the treatise and replaced its appendix on bladder size with one *"containing additional (hernia)   cases and observations ... and also ... Strictures on the Remarks of Reviewers."*

The new material includes cases from Mr Bransby Cooper at Guy's, a nephew of Sir Astley, showing that Stephens was maintaining old contacts.   Maybe even an influence of his late friend Keats (died 1821) can be discerned in his irritation with reviewers, for the new title-page proclaims a defiant quotation from Byron:
"Moved by a great example, I pursue,
     The self same road, and make my own review."
The   second edition appeared in 1831, the year Harriot died. Stephens had chosen a new publisher who also had connections with the Borough but its production seems not to have gone without a hitch.   Parts of the copy in the Wellcome Library appear to have identical typeface to the first edition but it contains both prefaces and both appendices. This copy, incidentally, was initially presented by Stephens to a Dr. Hope and its dedication, presumably in Stephens' hand, is written in ink which is still a bright blue (fig 5).

Stephens, the Medical Society of London and Cholera
The title page of the new edition tells us that Stephens is not only a MRCS, but also *"...one of the Council of   the Medical Society London"*. At this date this society (MSL) was a venerable and active association whose debates were topical, authoritative, widely reported and influential[16]. It was founded in 1773 and until 1850 it had its headquarters in Bolt Court on the north side of Fleet Street, not far via Blackfriars Bridge from Stamford Street.   Membership was by election so that patronage was necessary. It held weekly meetings on Tuesday nights throughout the year, with a four-month recess during the summer. These were mostly concerned with discussions on medical problems, and topics that led to a good debate could be continued at the next meeting.   Administrative business was discussed at intervals at extraordinary meetings, but more routine administration was left to a council most of whose members were elected annually. There was a social side to the society, and following the annual Commemorative meeting on 8 March, when annual reports were made and election results announced, members (93 of them in 1828) would retire to the London Coffee House in Ludgate Hill to dine convivially; one can guess that the memory of founder members was toasted more than once.

A

TREATISE

ON

OBSTRUCTED AND INFLAMED

HERNIA:

AND ON

MECHANICAL OBSTRUCTIONS

OF

THE BOWELS INTERNALLY.

SECOND EDITION.

WITH

An Appendix,

CONTAINING

ADDITIONAL CASES AND OBSERVATIONS,

Illustrated by Diagrams,

AND ALSO

STRICTURES ON THE REMARKS OF REVIEWERS.

Moved by a great example, I pursue
The self-same road, and make my own review.
LORD BYRON.

BY HENRY STEPHENS,

MEMBER OF THE ROYAL COLLEGE OF SURGEONS, AND ONE OF THE COUNCIL OF THE
MEDICAL SOCIETY OF LONDON.

London:

PUBLISHED BY S. HIGHLEY, 32, FLEET STREET,

AND WEBB STREET, MAZE POND, BOROUGH.

1831.

*(fig 5) Title Page of Stephens' HERNIA TREATISE
Second Edition,1831 with Inscription (Wellcome Library, London)*

14

Stephens may have attended society meetings as a guest in 1828, but he was elected as a member shortly after his marriage in September 1829 and he then attended fairly regularly, listed in the minutes among the surgeons[17]. He not only attended seventeen of the thirty meetings in 1830 but spoke in five discussions. He contributed on diverse topics including diseases of the joints, puerperal fever, brandy as a medicine, but especially on the subject of hernia. In his first speech (Nov 16, 1829), he described two cases of hernia in which, after the hernial protuberances had *"been returned the abdomen..."* there were still injurious adhesions between *"the hernial contents and the sac."* These cases seem very like those described in his book which had been very recently published. They were accepted rather dismissively by the meeting as being *"...very rare ..."*, and the book was not mentioned. The debate must have continued at another time, for later in the month (Nov 30, 1829) Stephens is on his feet quickly to dispel the impression that he had previously argued for a delay in operating on strangulated hernia. The chairman, the flamboyant and successful surgeon Thomas Calloway, emphatically confirmed the necessity of quick intervention for hernia before business moved on. This difference in emphasis between Stephens and Calloway concerning hernia treatment persisted to other occasions and surfaced for instance in a debate almost a year latter. But Stephens' attendance and conduct must have made a favourable impression on fellow members. He was elected a *"scrutator"* for society elections in 1830, and in 1831 and 1833-5 was annually elected to the society's Council.

The Council was responsible for most of the administrative affairs of the society: membership, subscriptions, finance, furniture and awards etc. They held about half a dozen meetings a year, but their minutes were so brief as not to identify individual contributions. They do record Stephens being put onto a committee that was to review the workings of the society's library in 1833. This project required reliability and activity as the library was a prized asset of the society and seems not to have been well managed. After better management it grew in reputation and value and its eventual sale in financially hard times provided a welcome source of income for essential building repairs[16].

Stephens was present at a meeting of the Society on November 28, 1831 when news arrived that cholera had reached England. A pandemic of the disease had been sweeping Asia and the Middle East for a year or so and had inevitably reached Europe and North America. A long and very diffuse letter had been received from James Hall RCS, a naval surgeon, concerning an outbreak of cholera among *"... his Majestys ships in Ordinary in the River Medway..."*

during the summer and autumn. A Secretary was instructed to make a summary of the paper as the discussion proceeded. Stephens was soon speaking and he described the case of a patient whose symptoms were very similar to those of Asiatic cholera and who was, for instance, producing *"rice-water stools"* somewhat resembling *"half dissolved blancmange"*. The patient survived, and this was attributed to energetic nursing including the application of blankets soaked in hot water and the administration of brandy and opium. The disease soon spread from the afflicted boats, and although Stephens could describe his first case in November, by next February, the President, Dr John Burke, could describe his first eight.

Later assessments showed that Stephens' area, Southwark and Lambeth, was very badly affected and that the disease was very virulent there. The seriousness of the situation probably explains why Stephens attended at least two meetings in December 1831 just before (5th) and after (19th) his daughter's death and burial in Redbourn (17th).

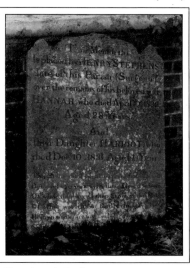

This Memorial
Is placed by HENRY STEPHENS
Late of this Parish (Surgeon).
Over the remains of his beloved wife
HANNAH, who died April 10th, 1832
Aged 28 Years
And
Their Daughter HARRIOT, who
Died Dec. 10th, 1831, Aged 1 Year
This stone shall speak no praise but only tell
How my heart mourns for those I loved so well.
Ah! while they lived I thought not of the bliss
Of other worlds, but fondly clung to this-
Heaven to attract my soul's high hopes above
Snatched both the bond and token of my love.

(fig 6)   GRAVESTONE St. Mary's Churchyard, Redbourn

Cholera was to be the main topic of Society debates for the next two years. Outside speakers were invited and many visitors attended. Aspects discussed included symptoms, contagiousness, medicines and even causes. Not all the debates were enlightening. It must be remembered that they were held almost twenty years before John Snow (1813-1858), later a distinguished President of the Society, removed the handle from the pump of the sewage-contaminated well in Broad Street, Soho, and demonstrated that the disease was water-borne; it was even longer (1884) before Robert Koch, at no little risk to his life, isolated the causative bacterium, *Vibrio comma*[17]. In 1832 suggested sources of the disease included miasmas, "unsound rice", and divine displeasure   and occasionally the audience was raised either to fury or laughter.   Proposed medicines were also various.

Late in 1831 Dr James Johnson had drawn attention to the efficacy of mercury on the (unlikely) grounds that it stimulated glandular secretions and that this would counteract the extreme dehydration that the disease produced. Attention soon turned to faster-acting compounds of mercury and Johnson eventually advocated blood-letting and doses of calomel. Stephens adopted calomel quickly but, like others, added small amounts of opium with it and according to his daughter [1] made some for "gratuitous distribution" in his neighbourhood; its efficacy acquired a reputation locally and also among local sailors engaged in cholera-prone voyages to Australia.

Martha Walsh[1], relying again on her father's recollections, also mentions that the *"heavy and incessant work and anxiety entailed during these two years affected the doctor's health very seriously. He had also lost his...wife...and little girl, which overwhelmed him with grief."* His life was feared for and his friend Mackereth, sent for in haste, was shocked at the state in which he found him. This episode probably occurred in the late summer of 1832, when, following his wife's death, he did not attend Society meetings from April to December. He may well have had a mild bout of cholera. In a later discussion on cholera symptoms at the Society (28 Oct., 1833) the secretary records Stephens's comments that:
"during the time of its [The Cholera's] prevailence, he had himself suffered from unusual rumblings in the Bowels, a threatening of Diarrhea, numbness of the limbs, occasional cramps, an alarmed state of mind, & coldness of the extremities; he believed that these symptoms lasted some time before the health broke, and that they might prevail to a great extent without a final attack of Cholera:...among other symptoms he ought to have mentioned affections of the heart, accompanied by a rapid & intermittent Pulse."

This self-diagnosis was met with some scepticism, but he was emphatic that his symptoms were genuine and not a consequence of apprehension. It is difficult to judge now whether he had been infected with cholera and had proved genuinely resistant or whether his infection was with an attenuated strain of bacteria; the remarkable resistance of some people to the disease was classically demonstrated in Munich in 1884, when Professor Pettenkoffer, a fierce sceptic of the great bacteriologist Robert Koch, drank with little effect a test-tube full of Koch's newly isolated *Vibrio comma* [18,19] ; there was enough vibrio, as Paul de Kruif [18] comments, *"..to infect a regiment."*

Cholera was not such a social menace in 1834 and Society minutes[17] were not written so comprehensively or so legibly. Stephens was still active in the Society and its Council. He was re-elected to Council in March 1835, but there is little evidence that he attended meetings. There is no doubt that his interest in medicine was being replaced by that of ink production during these years. But there is a postscript to his brushes with cholera.

GENERAL BOARD of HEALTH.

PRECAUTIONS

AGAINST

CHOLERA.

1. **Apply for Medicine immediately to stop Looseness of the Bowels, or it may bring on Cholera.**

2. Do not take any strong opening Medicine without Medical advice.

3. **Beware of Drink,** for excess in Beer, Wine, or Spirits is likely to be followed by Cholera.

4. Drink no Water which has not been boiled : and avoid that which is not quite clear and well tasted.

5. **Avoid** eating Meat that is tainted, decayed or unripe fruit, and stale Fish or raw vegetables. Cooked Vegetables, or ripe and cooked Fruit, in moderation, are a necessary part of diet at all times.

6. **Avoid** fasting too long : be moderate at Meals.

7. **Avoid** great fatigue, and getting heated and then chilled.

8. **Avoid** getting wet, or remaining in wet Clothes.

9. **Keep yourself clean**, and your body and feet as dry and as warm as your means and your occupation will permit.

10. **Keep your rooms well cleaned and lime-washed;** remove all dirt and impurities immediately.

11. Keep your windows open as much as possible to admit fresh air; and, if necessary, use Chloride of Lime or Zinc to remove any offensive smells.

12. If there are any dust, or dirt heaps, foul drains, bad smells, or other nuisances in the house or neighbourhood, make complaint without delay to the Local Authorities having legal power to remove them, or if there be no such authorities, or if you do not know who they are, complain to the Board of Guardians.

(fig 7) Typical CHOLERA Poster

During the two cholera years, 1832-33, Stephens had been making notes on the disease but had never completed them. However a further epidemic in 1848-9 re-awakened his interest and prompted him to publish a treatise on the matter. *Cholera: an analysis of its epidemic, and contagious character*, a tract of 47 pages, probably appeared first in 1848 and was reprinted in 1849 [20]. The preface emphasises the effect that the two tragic years had on him: *"The many tragic scenes then witnessed left impressions on my mind which have never been effaced... Two persons died in my house from it."* He confesses that by now *"I have seceded from the practice of medicine and have been engaged in other occupations,"* but *"... am anxious to make known and to communicate what I think may be serviceable to the Profession of which I am still a member, and to the cause of relieving human calamities and suffering."* The treatise recapitulates many of the views and opinions that had been expressed in the debates at the Medical Society of London. He describes incidents and specific cases that Martha Walsh later described anecdotally [1]. He argues that the best medicines for cholera treatment will be found amongst those chemicals that stimulate salivation and those such as tannins, barks and creosote which prevent the putrefaction of animal and vegetable matter. He especially recommends mercury derivatives and gives the recipe of the calomel-opium concoction which he prescribed and which originated from the Asiatic experience of doctors of the East India Company.

He seems unaware of the work of John Snow who was now a Vice President of MSL, for it was this epidemic that prompted Snow to remove the handle from the pump of the sewage-contaminated well in Broad Street, Soho, and led to his essay *On the Mode of Communication of Cholera* (1849) with its conclusion that the disease *"commences primarily in the alimentary canal and is due to swallowing morbid material from the excretions of victims, usually [in] drinking water"* [16]. Stephens' treatise must have been soon overshadowed by that of Snow. The copy now in the Wellcome Library was initially presented by Stephens to the library of the MSL, but its pages, uncut until recently, suggest that it had never been consulted.

Stephens' second marriage (1840)
In 1840, eight years after the death of Hannah, Stephens remarried. His new wife was Anne Reilly (O'Reilly), a 26-year-old spinster from Holborn. The marriage took place at the parish church of St Andrew, Holborn on 3 May and was witnessed by Samuel Josiah, Stephens' brother, and the brother and sister of the bride. This was the church

in which Stephens' parents were married and suggests that the Stephens family had not lost contact with friends in this area. Martha Walsh [1] describes Anne, her mother, as "...*beautiful with a face full of intelligence and feeling, joined to a rare elegance of form and grace of movement*", and she emphasizes her liberal ideas in politics and taste for literature and poetry. Martha is less flattering about Anne's father, Joseph Charles Reilly. She claims that he came from County Longford in Ireland to study law and train for the Bar, but he is described on the marriage certificate as a jeweller. She describes him as "...*selfish, harsh, neglectful of everything but his own comfort. No one ever had a good word to say of him.*" Whatever his qualities, his children seem more urbane. Anne has some cosmopolitan style, and her honeymoon-like holiday was spent in Brussels, and later, with the help of her French-speaking sister Ellen, had her two eldest children, Henry Charles (b. 1841) and Martha (b. 1843) educated in Paris.

Ink Manufacture

Sometime soon after the traumatic years 1832-3, Stephens' attention was increasingly drawn to the poor quality of the writing inks available to him, whether they were obtained commercially or were home-made. Maybe it was initially just an interest that diverted his attention from more depressing family matters. One can speculate that he was already familiar with ink-making from his childhood in Redbourn, as there was a strong tradition of domestic ink-making in rural areas, and many recipes using available nuts, barks and berries have survived from the 16th to the 19th centuries in domestic note-books, recipe books and diaries [21, 22]. But anyway, his interest in the chemical aspects of the process and his ability to experiment had almost certainly been encouraged by the influence of Dr Alex Marcet during his time at Guy's [6].

> To make common Inke of wine take a quart
> Two ounces of Gumme let that be a part,
> Five ounces of Gals, of Copres take three,
> Long standing doth make it the better to be.
> If wine ye do want, rain water is best,
> And then as much stuffe as aboue at the least.
> If Inke be too thicke, put vinegar in:
> For water doth make the colour more dim.

(fig 8)   *Typical "INKE" recipe from the 17th century*

Moreover his familiarity with the malting and brewing activities of his parents may have given him an insight into the management of small-scale factory operations. It is not known how far his interest in ink was affected by the close proximity to his house in Stamford Street of the Clowes printing works, reputedly the largest steam-driven printing works in the world, employing by the end of the 1830s some 600 workers [14,15].

His experiments and small-scale manufacturing started in the cellars of 54 Stamford Street, but were soon moved a few hundred yards along the street to a *"yard, stable, workshop and shed"* where he had formerly kept his doctor's horse and carriage. This rented site, measuring 57 x 65 feet, was reached from an entrance in Princes Street (now Coin Street) and so was adjacent to Clowes' printing works [23]. Here he employed a *"...foreman and men bottling and so forth..."* [1]. The foreman may have been Ebenezer Nash who was a partner in the manufacturing patent that Stephens took out in 1837; the patent [24] describes Nash as a tallow chandler from Buross Street in the parish of St George-in-the-East, but the census of 1851 records him as "chemical color and ink maker" living near the factory in Duke Street just off Stamford Street. Stephens' approach to the manufacturing project was, in spite of initial discouragement from his brother and colleagues, well organised and energetic. Walsh [1] tells how her father market-researched his inks on his friends before launching them onto the public, and of his persistence in overcoming production bottlenecks, and his speed in establishing agents in France and the USA. Musgrove [23] lists successive moves of manufacturing location as the business grew; some, but not all of the production moved out to Grove House in Finchley when Stephens moved his family there, and it remained there during Stephens' life-time.

Stephens' formulation of inks and wood-stains was essentially traditional. His celebrated blue-black ink was a *"tanno-gallate of iron dissolved in sulphate of indigo"* [23, 21]. Inks made from the mineral iron sulphate (green copperas) and gallic acid and its derivatives, usually extracted from the insect-induced galls of Mediterranean oak trees, had been used since the twelfth century, and had formed the basis of the endurable script of medieval manuscripts; indigo, an extract of plants such as the woad plant (*Isatis tinctoria*) had also been one of the many natural colourants used in different writing fluids since ancient times [21]. His skill seems to have been in formulating them together in the correct proportions and being meticulous about the quality of the ingredients he used. The indigo in the mixture gives an immediate blue colour to the script on the surface of the paper and allows the iron gallate to penetrate into the paper before the iron is oxidized from the ferrous to the ferric state causing the formation of an insoluble black precipitate bound within the fibres of the paper [21, 23].

This formulation, probably containing some gum Arabic to decrease premature formation of the black precipitate, gives the ink a longer shelf life, and it also avoids excesses of acid or iron which are deleterious to both metal pen nibs and paper. Another of the "*Writing Fluids*" that he formulated and marketed, his "*Patent Unchangeable Blue Fluid*" almost certainly contained Prussian Blue. This material had been used by other ink producers [21], and its purification is partly the subject of one of Stephens' patents.

The precise recipes for Stephens' inks seem not to be known; it may be that they are still the confidential property of the commercial inheritors of the Stephens Ink Company. The two patents registered in his name do not resolve the matter. The first was taken out in 1837 [24], in the last few months of the reign of King William IV, in the names of Henry Stephens of Charlotte Street in the parish of Saint Marylebone and of Ebenezer Nash of Buross Street in the parish of St George-in-the-East, Middlesex. Its registered description, "*Certain Improvements in Manufacturing Colouring Matter, and rendering Certain Colour or Colours Applicable to Dyeing, Staining and Writing*", was slightly modified five months later to include the word "*more*" before "*Applicable to*". It claims patent rights on four procedures; first, a method for recovering salts of prussic acid from nitrogenous gases evolved during the distillation of a mixture of animal material and alkali, by passing the gases directly into hot, concentrated alkali; second, the use of strong acids to digest the dye, Prussian blue, to render it more soluble in oxalic acid and the use of oxalic acid as a solvent for Prussian blue in preparing inks and stains; third, the use of oxalate and its derivatives as solvents for cochineal and other red dyes; fourth, mixing carbonaceous materials such as lamp black suspended in alkaline solutions of resins, with coloured solutions to make indelible coloured inks.

While suggesting some components of the five major inks that Stephens manufactured, the patent gives no clear recipes. The patent does indicate however the hazardous and industrial nature of Stephens' chemical activities, especially if they included the production of Prussian blue by the alkaline incineration of animal material and it is surprising that they were carried out in 1837 in cramped, residential premises. It suggests a high degree of care and organisation by Stephens. The other patent was also registered in 1837 [26] solely in Stephens' name and giving his own address in Stamford Street rather than that of his brother Samuel Josiah in Charlotte Street. It concerns inkstands and pens rather than ink. It claims patent rights for the design of a stopper for "fountain" inkstands, and a method of moulding pens from natural horns, bones and shells by pressing them in heated metal dies. Stephens' interest in writing extended from inks themselves to their proper storage and their behaviour on pens during writing.

The virtues of Stephens' inks and inkstands were forcefully advocated by Wm Baddiley in the *Mechanics' Magazine* in 1836 [27] even before the inkstands had their patent stopcocks. His long, detailed letter concludes
"I have received much personal convenience from the use of Mr Stephens' writing fluid; and have much pleasure in thus publicly expressing my thanks for the same. Wishing him every success..."
He clearly had either contact with Stephens or access to his writings, and quotes him twice. These show that Stephens was well aware of what can go wrong with inks that had too much iron, but they give no specific details of his recipes and are couched in the limited chemical understanding of the time. Baddeley judges Stephens to have been *"eminently fortunate"* in the substances used for his inks and commends his "minute attention" to their proportions and their purity. He notes, as a measure of their success *"... that imitators and adulterators have sprung up, like mushrooms..."*

Over a hundred years later, another commentator[28] quotes a contemporary (but unspecified) newspaper article that praises the same blue-black ink and its waterproof qualities. *"Its permanence is proved by the fact that its legibility was not impaired by three months under the sea in the shipwrecked Oregon. Other documents that were recovered from the shipwrecked SS Egypt after eight years were read easily; The Treaty of Versailles was signed in this ink"*. This last comment emphasises the use of this ink as a government-approved "ink of record"; throughout the 19th and 20th centuries administrators of many countries had realised that important legal documents had over the last few hundred years been written in inferior inks which had faded.

Following a Prussian initiative in 1878 [21] many countries had introduced specifications and standards of permanence for inks used for government purposes. Stephens' blue-black ink clearly complied with these requirements and had been accepted as such by the participants to the Treaty of Versailles. Mitchell [21] gives excerpts from *British Specifications for the Supply of Writing Inks, Ink Powders and Ink Concentrates to H.M. Stationery Office* (1934). The apparently water-resistant qualities of Stephens' blue-black ink would doubtless have recommended its use to governments. These agencies could not rely on the intervention of St Cuthbert to preserve their records as did the monks of Lindisfarne when their celebrated Gospels were lost at sea sometime in the eighth century [21].

In summary, two characteristics contributed to the success of Stephens' blue-black ink. First, unlike traditional iron-tannate inks, it was not over-exposed to the atmosphere during manufacture to convert these compounds into black insoluble particles that would remain on the surface of the paper; thus the oxidation of ferrous compounds to insoluble ferric forms would take place within the fibres of the paper to which it was applied. Second, the addition of indigo gave an added intensity of colour on first application to paper. In spite of an earlier claim that Stephens was initially responsible for the first of these innovations [29], Mitchell's later authoritative review of inks [21] makes it clear that both un-oxidised inks and indigo inks had been suggested and tried in the late eighteenth century. But he recognised that Stephens was using such formulations in 1836 even though the earliest patent specifically for them was made by Leonhardi in Hanover in 1856. So although Stephens was not the *fons et origo* of this formulation of blue-black ink, he was one of a group of pioneers and certainly the most successful of them in its commercialisation.

The Finchley connection
In the early 1840s Stephens' family was growing but so was his income. There seemed little need for him to remain in crowded Southwark and he must have felt able to taste the delights of a country gentleman's life. By 1844 he had bought and renovated a rambling old house, Grove House, in Ballards Lane, Finchley [23].

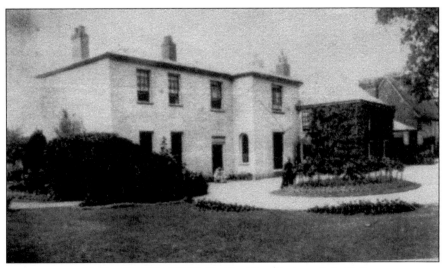

(fig 9)   GROVE HOUSE, Finchley (The Stephens Collection)

24

Finchley was then a small very rural village about six miles north of London's Regents Park. It was close enough to London for Stephens to attend to his business activities there and to join in metropolitan cultural life. The village also gave easy access to Hertfordshire and his relatives, and he may well have first become acquainted with it on horseback journeys from Redbourn to Southwark. The house had a large garden and *three good fields at the back, and three more just across the road, called the "front fields"*. It provided, Stephens' daughter affirms [1], *" a most delightful life for children, hay making, blackberrying, etc, plenty of pets... We had cows, horses, pigs, and later, first a donkey and then a pony."* There was even *"..a pet deer that would walk quietly by father's side through the village."*

There was plenty of room in this idyll for family additions. These were Catherine (1846), Harold (1848), Ellen (1853) and Julian (1855). As the house was halfway between Uncle Josiah's farm near Barnet and his town house in Marylebone there were frequent visits from cousins. Stephens seems to have taken much care with his children's education, and in 1850, encouraged by his sister-in-law Ellen, the two eldest children, Henry Charles and Martha, spent two years at school in Paris learning French. This experience seems to have been successful according to Martha's account, and even the Parisian *coup d'état* of December 1851 only caused a *frisson*. He took especial care of Henry Charles' chemical education after he had finished at University College School, and in a suitably equipped outhouse in the garden, instructed him in the manufacture of inks and stains. He took him to hear Faraday's popular lectures at the Royal Institution in London. He clearly expected the boy to enter the family business and succeed him in due course. In this effort, he was extraordinarily successful. Not only did Henry Charles develop the company, but continued the benevolent connection with Finchley that is still commemorated by the Finchley Society and their Stephens Collection museum in Avenue House in East End Road.

Stephens threw himself into village affairs becoming a churchwarden, attending vestry meetings and lecturing on electricity in the village schoolroom. He rode with the local hunts and kept some fine greyhounds. His social life extended well beyond the village and with his wife he continually attended annual meetings of the Social Science Congress in one or another of the country's big towns. He cultivated old and new friendships, such as that with Sir B.W. Richardson [8]. He must have visited his factories and offices frequently and was assiduous in defending his patent rights against infringement. A particularly troublesome infringement involved Morrell & Co, ink manufacturers. Martha Walsh describes it as stressful and expensive but gives few details. The census of 1861 gives a snapshot of Stephens' household at the height of this active and enjoyable life. Besides Henry, now 64 years old, and Anne, there are six children between six and twenty years, Aunt Ellen, Sarah and Matilda Hands, a cook and housemaid respectively, and two labourers, one of whom worked in the Colour Factory.

The family's social life involved a continual contact with the Mackereth family living in the environs of Hull. The friendship between the two ex-medical students was enduring, but new ones developed. There was a business connection between George Mackereth and Samuel Josiah Stephens [30], but more important, a romantic attachment between 22-year-old Henry Charles and the younger (21-year-old) Margaret Agnes Mackereth. This met with the approval and probably blessings of all concerned and they were married in the Parish church of Keyingham, East Yorks, on 28 April in 1863. *"We all went down to be present"*, wrote Martha,[1] *"also Uncle Josiah and Aunt Mary Anne, my father in good health and spirits, with my mother"*. Martha, as well as six other sisters of the bride and groom, witnessed the signing of the certificate. The large wedding party may well have travelled to Yorkshire by rail; with the little inconvenience of a few changes such a journey from St Pancras station was possible in 1863.

The developing railway system played another active role in Stephens' life, and also witnessed its last, tragic moments. The Metropolitan Railway opened its three-mile, semi-underground track from Paddington to Farringdon Street in London in January 1863 with trains running every fifteen minutes during the working day. This provided a convenient way for Stephens to cross London to the city after a short horse-drawn journey from Finchley to Paddington. He may have been one of its early users and used it frequently for the next 17 months after the wedding. He used it for the last time on 15 September 1864 when he and Henry Charles had been to the city on unspecified business. The station superstructure was much like it is at present but the atmosphere smokier [31]. Stephens must have had some difficulty as they struggled with the crowd onto the platform for the return journey, and to help him, his son relieved him of his bag and overcoat [1]. But the men lost contact in the crowd, and Henry Charles boarded the train thinking that his father was already on board. He was not, and had presumably collapsed on the platform. Walsh [1] describes the anxiety and confusion of the evening and night, with expeditions sent from Finchley and Uncle Josiah's house, to trace Henry. But it was not until the next morning that his body was located.

He was buried in St Marylebone Cemetery, Finchley, where a solid monument still commemorates him as well as other members of his family .

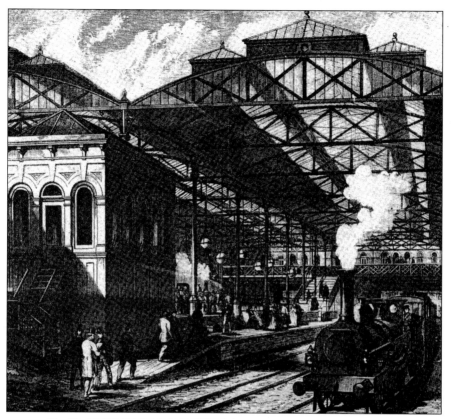

(fig 10) *FARRINGDON ROAD STATION, 1866 (London Transport Collection)*

His widow Anne continued to live in Grove House with her unmarried daughter Ellen and, for sometime, her son Julian, until her death in 1895. Julian called himself a *cupras merchant* in a Census return, and probably worked for the family ink company; but the real control of this company lay firmly in the hands of Henry Charles who lived with his family in some style in nearby Avenue House until he died in 1918.[23,30] In his hands, it flourished well into the next century.

References: Henry Stephens

1   Walsh, M. (1925) *The Life of Henry Stephens F.R.C.S.* The Stephens Collection, Avenue House, Finchley, N3 3QE.

2   Featherstone, A. (2001) *Redbourn's History.* Redbourn Books.

3   Pierpoint, W.S. (2008) *Markyate Doctors and their Redbourn Pupil.* Markyate's Past. 17, pp. 2-5. (Journal of Markyate Local History Society, ISSN 0963-3901)

4   Gittings, R. (1971) *John Keats.*   Penguin Books: Harmondsworth, Middlesex.

5   Motion, A. (1997) *Keats.* Faber & Faber Ltd. London.

6   South, J. F. (1884) *Memorials.* (Ed. C.L. Fentoe). John Murray, Albemarle Street, London.

7   Leaback, D.H. (2000) *Re-weaving Rainbows.* Authentica Publications, Biolink Technology Ltd. (Tel. 01923 854624)

8   Richardson, B.W. (1884) *An Esculapian Poet - John Keats. The Asclepiad.* Vol 1 , part 2, April 1884. (Published by Sir Benjamin Ward Richardson, M.D., F.R.S.; London.)

9   Colvin, S. (1917) *John Keats.* Macmillan and Co. Ltd. London.

10   Rollins, H.E. (1948) Ed. *The Keats Circle*, vol 2.   Harvard University Press, Cambridge, Mass. USA.

11   Stephens, H. (1831) *A Treatise on Obstructed and Inflamed Hernia: and on Mechanical Obstructions of the Bowels Internally.* 2nd Edition. S. Highley, 32 Fleet Street, London. (Copy in Wellcome Library for the History of Medicine, London)

12   Such, R. (2005) *The Inns and Public Houses of Redbourn* Privately published. pp. 64. Available from Redbourn Village Museum, The Common, Redbourn, Herts AL3 7NB.

13   Stephens, H. (1997) *Journal of an Excursion into the North, November 1827.* Edited by Jennifer Stephens. Published by The Stephens Collection, Avenue House, Finchley.

14   Renier, H. (2006) *Lambeth Past.* Historical Publications Ltd., London.

15   Clowes, W.B. (1953) *Family Business*, 1803-1953. William Clowes and Sons Ltd, Little New Street, London.

16   Hunting, P. (2003) *The Medical Society of London, 1773-2003.* Medical Society of London, London.

17   *Medical Society of London: Minutes of General and of Council Meetings*; microfilms, cat. no. WMS/MF4: the Wellcome Library, Euston Rd, London.

18   De Kruif, Paul (1926) *Microbe Hunters.* Harcourt, Brace Inc, New York.

19   Henrici, A.T. and Ordal E.J. (1948) *The Biology of Bacteria.* D.C. Heath & Company, London.

20   Stephens, H. (1849)   *Cholera: an analysis of its epidemic, endemic and contagious character etc.*   Henry Renshaw, London.   In Bound Tracts, MST.326.10. Wellcome History of Medicine Library, London.

21   Mitchell, C. A.   (1937)   *Inks: Their Composition and Manufacture.* Charles Griffin & Co. London.

22   Nickell, J. (1990)   *Pen, Ink and Evidence: A Study of Writing and Writing Materials* for the Penman, Collector, and Document Detective. The University Press of Kentucky, Lexington, USA.

23   Musgrove, P. (1984)   *Henry C. Stephens: An Avenue House Centenary.* The Finchley Society, Avenue House, Finchley, London.

24   Patent No. 7342 (1837) *Manufacture of Colouring Matters for Dying, Staining and Writing. 18 October 1837.* Business and Patents Information Services, 3rd Floor Suite, Central Library, Calverley St, Leeds LS1 3AB.

25   Encyclopaedia Britannica (1910). *Ink.* Eleventh Edition, vol 14, pp. 571-573. Cambridge University Press, Cambridge.

26   Patent No 7333. (1837). *Inkstands and Pens. 28 September 1837.* Business and Patents Information Services, 3rd Floor Suit, Central Library, Calverley St., Leeds LS1 3AB.

27 Baddeley,W. (1836) *Stephens' Improved Fountain Inks.* Mechanics' Magazine, No. 673, Letters, July 2nd.

28 Walker, M. (1960) *Redbourn.* Privately published, p. 76.

29 Mitchell, C.A. & Hepworth, T.C. (1924) *Inks: Their Composition and Manufacture.* Third Edition. Charles Griffin and Co., London.

30 Pierpoint, W.S. (This script). *Unparallel Lives... Part 3, George Wilson Mackereth.*

31 Lee, C.E. (1972). *The Metropolitan Line.* London Transport, 55 Broadway, Westminster, S.W.1.

JOHN KEATS (1795-1821)

POET

John Keats is a major figure in the literary landscape of the English-speaking world. As he hoped and possibly foresaw, he has joined "the immortals". He has attracted countless lectures, articles and biographies. Biographers have been well aware that he was a qualified doctor even though he never practised [1,2,3,4]. It would be presumptuous for this writer to try to contribute seriously to the literature devoted to him. All that is attempted here is a brief summary of some aspects of his life where it either intertwined with those of his fellow medical students, Henry Stephens and George Wilson Mackereth, or where it invites comparison with their lives.

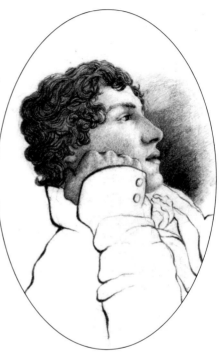

(fig 11)   Pencil drawing of JOHN KEATS by CHARLES ARMITAGE BROWN, 1819 (National Portrait Gallery, London)

Background

He was born somewhere in the city of London in 1795, and baptised at the church of St Botolph's Without (Bishopsgate) on December 18. His father, Thomas Keats (1773-1804) was an ostler or principal servant at the Swan and Hoop, a large inn on The Pavement, Moorgate, close to London Wall on the then eastern edge of London. His mother, Frances (1775-1810), was the daughter of John and Alice Jennings who owned the leasehold on the inn. Thomas and his family lived in Craven Street, about three-quarters of a mile north of the Swan and Hoop, and it was here that Keats' three brothers, George (1797), Tom (1799) and the short-lived Edward (1801-1802) were born. But in 1802, the Jennings, Frances' parents, retired from running the inn, and while still retaining its lease went to live in rural Ponders End, some ten miles further north.

Thomas and Frances were invited to take over management of the inn at a rent of £44 a year. They accepted and moved their family into the upstairs accommodation that year. Settling in above the busy inn must have involved some upheaval which was aggravated by the death of young Edward, but there seems no reason to believe that the experience was traumatic to Keats. But more adjustments were necessary next year as a new baby, Fanny (Frances Mary), was born, and Keats with his brother George were sent as boarding-pupils to Clarke's school in Enfield. This school had a good reputation and was run on liberal and non-conformist principles by the enlightened John Clarke, who with his son Charles Cowden Clarke proved to be extraordinarily sympathetic and encouraging to Keats, encouraging in due course his acquaintance with the classical poets.

The boys were homesick at first but received frequent, reassuring visits from both parents and nearby grandparents. However, one of these visits was to result in a tragedy with far reaching effects. Thomas Keats came by himself to visit his boys on 15 April 1804. On the way home he stopped for a late supper at Southgate and on leaving he fell or was thrown from his horse, receiving head injuries from which he died the next day. Soon after his funeral, his distraught wife, presumably with baby Fanny, disappeared completely, leaving the inn and the boys to the care of relatives. She reappears after a few weeks but in June she remarried, in the church

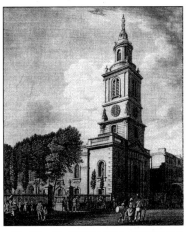

(fig 12)   St BOTOLPH'S WITHOUT (BISHOPSGATE)
(Keats House Hampstead, London)

where she had married Thomas, a young stranger, William Rawlings. Much has been written on the character of Frances and on her state of mind at this time, but worse was to come. Her father, John Jennings, died in March of the following year, leaving a substantial will mostly derived from his earnings at the Swan and Hoop.

Although Frances was a beneficiary she felt that she and her children had been poorly treated and she contested the will against her relatives. This led to interminable court transactions and to money wrangles that helped to tear the family apart. It also split Frances' relationship with Rawlings completely, and for the second time she ran away from the inn to live in unknown, possible degrading circumstances elsewhere. Rawlings was left to manage the inn by himself until its lease ran out, and after disposing of the lease he too left the area, disappearing from recorded history. Grandmother Alice, who had looked after John and George in school vacations, moved house from Ponders End to Edmonton within two miles of Enfield. She had no choice now but to take full responsibility for all her grandchildren, even though she was a 69-year-old widow.

This confused family life must have had a disturbing effect on John. For the next three years, he continued his education at Clarke's school. The Clarkes, especially Charles Cowden who was eight years older than John, were a stabilising influence on him, but he was prone to fits of temper and his behaviour was occasionally erratic. The next long crisis came in early 1809 when, after an absence of over three years, his mother reappeared. She must have presented a pathetic sight as she cautiously approached her own mother, asking whether she might return to live with her children again. She was accepted. But she was a broken woman, wearied, depressed and ill; apart from rheumatism she was showing signs of the tuberculosis that had recently claimed her brother and which was so cruelly to overshadow John's life. She was accepted into her mother's household more as a patient than a guest.

There had always been a strong bond between son and mother and this seems to have been intensified in the new circumstances. Keats *"appointed himself her principal nurse, caring for her with a passionate possessiveness... He sat up whole nights in a great chair, would suffer nobody to give her medicine but himself, and even cooked her food; ...and read novels to her in her intervals of ease."* [2] This intense nursing continued in the school holidays until March 1810 when Frances died of tuberculosis. It had a profound effect on John. It galvanised his studies at school, especially of the poets, turning him from an inattentive pupil to an obsessional, hard-working, prize-winning student. This continued after his mother's death. Andrew Motion suggests that as well as energising him this period had a lasting effect on him, emphasising, among other things, the connection between literature and healing. This would not only inform much of his poetry but it might well have influenced his entry into the medical profession.

Medical Apprenticeship
In autumn 1810, about six months after his mother's death, Keats left Clarke's school and entered an apprenticeship with Thomas Hammond of Edmonton. Suggestions that he was forced into this arrangement either by his well-meaning grandmother or by Richard Abbey, the newly appointed trustee and future guardian of the Keats children, seem unlikely. The evidence suggests that Keats was not unhappy about it. In spite of the ups and downs of the arrangement

the next five years have often been described as *"the most placid period of his painful life"* [1]. Certainly the arrangement kept him close to Cowden Clarke, whom he visited more than weekly, and kept him near to his grandmother who lived until December 1814.

Thomas Hammond was a respected figure in Edmonton society, coming from a medical family which had been practising there for at least three generations. He was a neighbour and friend of the Jennings family having attended Keats' grandparents and mother as well as patients at Clarke's school. His surgery was a cottage in his garden above which was a cramped attic which was Keats' sleeping quarters. Keats would take most of his meals in the doctor's house, where, in a sense he replaced Hammond's own son who was apprenticed to another doctor.

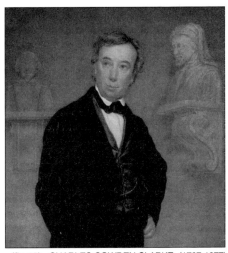

(fig 13) CHARLES COWDEN CLARKE (1787-1877) (Artist unknown c.1834 National Portrait Gallery, London)

Keats' duties would have been very similar to those of Henry Stephens in Markyate [5], graduating from more menial housekeeping to those of a skilled nurse and midwife. But the domestic atmosphere could not have been so comfortably relaxed as those experienced by Stephens.

Some time after his grandmother's death there occurred a poorly described incident that may have led to threatening behaviour and clenched fists between apprentice and either his master or his master's son. This seems to have led to Keats leaving his lodgings with Hammond and seeking separate accommodation, possibly in Edmonton and with his brother Tom. This did not ease Keats' strained financial situation, but it did not break his apprenticeship nor completely destroy trust. Hammond had been trained at Guy's Hospital and still maintained his contact with it. It was probably his guidance, testimony and even patronage that introduced Keats to the joint teaching hospitals of St Thomas' and Guy's where he could receive the training that was recently required of aspiring doctors by the Apothecary Act of 1815.

This is not the place to stress that this period of medical apprenticeship was, for Keats, the beginning of what could be regarded as his longer apprenticeship to literature and poetry. His frequent visits to the Clarkes, especially to Charles Cowden whose tutorage and access to a comprehensive library not only helped to stabilise him after the traumatic disruption of his family life, but introduced him to the culture that was to nurture and develop his latent genius [1,2].

Training in St Thomas' and Guy's Hospitals.

Keats may have been more familiar with London than either Stephens or Mackereth. But it must still have been a big change from rural Edmonton to crowded, slummy Southwark. He commented on the Borough's *"...jumbled heap of murky buildings..."* and described its street scene as a *"beastly place in dirt, turnings and windings."*[1,2] The squalid aspects of the area are ably described by Keats' biographers; Hannah Renier's illustrated history describes the same squalor of neighbouring Lambeth as well as the vigorous industrial enterprises that developed in the area [6].

The teaching hospitals must also have been dirty, crowded and distressing places even by contemporary standards, although, as we have commented, the teaching staff were of a very high quality, both professionally and educationally. Keats registered at Guy's on 1 October 1815, some days before either Stephens or Mackereth, and the next day paid the £25-4s necessary to become a surgical pupil. He seems to have had some recommendation or patronage that attracted the attention of Sir Astley Cooper, the surgeon who was the most celebrated and charismatic of his tutors. Cooper entrusted Keats to the care of two junior colleagues, George Cooper and Frederick

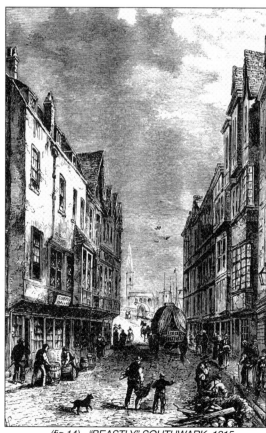

(fig 14)   "BEASTLY" SOUTHWARK, 1815

Tyrrell, and they quickly got him accommodation in their own nearby lodgings at 28 St Thomas Street, the house of a tallow-chandler called Markham, where he could share a common sitting room with them. He may well have been established here before Stephens and Mackereth came to occupy rooms on another floor of the house where they shared a second sitting room [7,8]. They too had registered at Guy's on the 14th and 4th of October. They must have become acquainted with Keats as they settled into the busy routine of lectures but this acquaintance intensified around Christmas when both Cooper and Tyrrell left Guy's, and as Stephens recollected in 1847 *"...John Keats, being alone, & to avoid the expense of having a sitting room to himself, asked to join us, which we readily agreed to. We were therefore constant Companions..."* [8].

The busy schedule of lectures, ward attendances and anatomical dissections that was the long daily routine of the students has been summarised earlier [5], and described fully in a contemporary source [7] and elsewhere [1,2]. So also has the comradery that it produced among the students, and the amusements and diversions that occupied their leisure. Keats fell easily into the company of *"...the more average type of medical student..."* [1] after losing the protective attentions of Cooper and Tyrrell. But the latter recollections of Stephens [8] indicate that he did not integrate completely. He seems to have been a little aloof and was vocal in his unpopular belief that studying medicine was an inferior occupation to studying poetry and that his own taste and ability in this direction were superior. *"... It may readily be imagined that this feeling was accompanied with a good deal of Pride and some conceit, and that amongst mere Medical students, he would walk, & talk as one of the Gods might be supposed to do, when mingling with mortals. This pride had exposed him, as may be readily imagined, to occasional ridicule, & some mortification..."* [8]

Other activities and habits of Keats also irritated Stephens and his colleagues. These include his apparent inattention to lectures, when he would readily fall into reveries or *"...scribble some doggerel rhymes..."* either in his own notes or *"...particularly if he got hold of another Students Syllabus"*. The paper cover of one of Stephens' own notebooks was not immune from this vandalism and was adorned with a fragment beginning
> *" Give me Women, Wine and Snuff*
> *Until I cry out "hold, enough !*
> *You may do so, sans objection*
> *Till the day of resurrection;*
> *For, bless my beard, they aye shall be*
> *My beloved Trinity. "*

This book cover is now carefully preserved in Trinity College,

Cambridge [8], but, understandably, the doggerel was never published by Keats [9].

Some of Keats' behaviour may, perhaps simplistically, be understood as a result of insecurity caused by his broken home life; it was interpreted by his colleagues, the "*mere medical students*", as arrogance and posturing. Their attitude may also have been tinged with envy. After only four weeks he was given the role of "dresser" or assistant to a surgeon, a post usually reserved for more senior students. This role was a mixed blessing as it was not, overall, of financial advantage to Keats and it meant extra work. Moreover his surgeon, William Lucas junior, appears not to have been the most skilful of his profession, and left Keats with some difficult clinical messes to tidy up. Keats seems to have coped with these situations very well, confirming Stephens' judgement of his being quick to learn. Nevertheless the post carried some prestige that others could envy.

Another source of envy was the apparent ease with which he passed his apothecary's licentiate examination (LSA) at the first try in July, 1816. Both Stephens and Mackereth failed their first attempts and only succeeded at retakes some eight months later. Keats never sat for his surgical examination as Stephens and Mackereth did, having decided during 1816 that he would dedicate himself to poetry; one can guess that had he sat, after his experience as a dresser, he would have been successful.

Another circumstance that set Keats apart from his fellows was that he had another social and intellectual life outside medical studies. His brothers lived in the city and were frequent visitors to St Thomas Street, often irritating his friends with their idolisation of him. Through his brother George he was introduced to poetic circles centred on the Mathew family, one of whom, George Felton Mathew, stimulated his enthusiasm if not his taste [2] and was later to elicit Stephens' recollections of Keats [8]. More importantly, Charles Cowden Clarke introduced him to Leigh Hunt, the radical journalist, publisher and man of letters

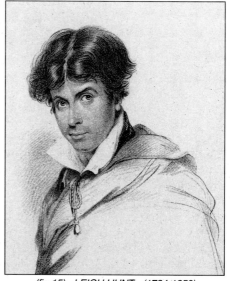

(fig 15) LEIGH HUNT (1784-1859)
Engraving of a drawing by J Hayter

whose arrest and imprisonment for his anti-government articles was a *cause célèbre* for the political left.

Hunt was a major influence in Keats' career, publishing his early poems and introducing him in due course to his circle of friends including Wordsworth, Shelley, Lamb, Hazlitt and other "immortals". His publication of Keats' *"O Solitude"* in May 1816, and his own essay on *"Three Young Poets"* in the December issue of the *Examiner,* confirmed Keats' resolution to dedicate his life to poetry rather than medicine, to make *"Poetry...the zenith of all his Aspirations"* as Stephens wrote. It is still unclear whether Keats' decision was also influenced by a growing dislike of surgery, especially the clumsy surgery of William Lucas.

Keats communicated this decision to his guardian Abbey, in a confrontation later paraphrased [2].
"Not intend to be a surgeon ! Why what do you mean to be ?
I mean to rely on my Abilities as a Poet.
John, you are either mad or a Fool, to talk in so absurd a Manner.
My mind is made up, said the youngster very quietly. I know that I possess Abilities greater than most Men, and therefore I am determined to gain my Living by exercising them.
Seeing nothing to be done Abbey called him a Silly Boy, & prophesied a speedy Termination to his inconsiderate Enterprise."

Nothing could be done. By November 1816, Keats had left St Thomas Street, and after a short spell in nearby Dean Street, was living with George and Tom in Cheapside in the city. He was more removed from his medical colleagues and his responsibilities at the hospital but nearer his poetic friend in Hampstead. He was now 21, had come into his own inheritance and his immediate dependence on Abbey was apparently broken. But Abbey was still the guardian of his siblings: sister Fanny would be in lodgings with him, with some degree of resentment, after she left school.

While the release from Abbey's authority gave Keats the freedom to develop his life in poetry, it deprived him of an influence which might have given him financial advice. Keats spent money freely and generously when he had it but seemed incapable of its long-term management. It is suggested that the experience of his mother's misguided attempts at lawsuits that split her family apart may have given him a morbid distaste for financial matters; it seems an avoidable misfortune for him that he never recognised and reclaimed an inheritance from his father, then held in Chancery, that brother George discovered two years after John's death [1,2].

Keats' connections with Guy's withered slowly and in a perfunctory way; he never took his surgical examination. In early 1817, as a protégé of both Hunt and the painter Haydon, he was assimilating the new artistically exalted society in which he now moved . The probable high point of this activity came at the end of this year (Dec 28) when he would dine in intimacy at Haydon's house in company with William Wordsworth, Thomas Monkhouse, and Charles Lamb[1,2]. The dinner took place in the painting studio of Haydon underneath the vast, as yet unfinished canvas of *Christ's Entry into Jerusalem*. In this picture the portraits of Wordsworth and Keats had been painted into the crowd as had those of Voltaire, Newton, Hazlitt and other luminaries. These images as well as the wine inspired a sparkling conversation so that the "immortal" dinner was long remembered in spite of its fatuous comments on Newton and natural philosophy (science), and their infamous toast to the "confusion of mathematics". But contact with his medical student friends slowly ceased.

We have commented on Stephens' visit to Keats (early 1817) when he lived with his brothers in Cheapside, and was struggling with the epic *Endymion*. We also noted their last meeting in Redbourn (June 22, 1818) as Keats was escorting George and his new wife to the emigration docks in Liverpool.

Stephens' memoir suggests that this might not have been Keats' first visit to this Hertfordshire village. *"After the period of our Studies were finished, at the Hospitals we saw little more of each other. He once went into the Country with me on a visit to my friends and stopped a day or two. He did not generally make the most favourable impression on people where he visited. He could not well unbend himself & was rather of an unsocial disposition, unless he was among those who were of his own tastes, & who would flatter him."*

The context suggests that this awkward occasion, possibly a visit to Stephens' family at the *Bull Inn*, may have occurred some time after his graduation and before their final meeting. Stephens cannot be accused of belonging to those who "would flatter" Keats, and this makes his critical comments all the more reliable. If he sounds a little grumpy in these memoirs, it is worth remembering that the script had been badgered out of him by George Felton Mathew.

Mathew had been friendly with Keats before he went to Guy's and St Thomas', and within his limits had encouraged Keats' poetic efforts and provided a social environment. But by 1847 Mathew had fallen on hard times[8]. He was a clerk to the Poor Law Commissioners and had a family of twelve to support. Some disagreement with the

Commissioners had led to his dismissal and eventual reinstatement at a lower level. He was desperate to secure the support of Richard Monkton Milnes, later Lord Houghton, in his cause, and as Milnes was collecting biographical material on Keats, Mathew had undertaken to get recollections from Stephens for him. There is a hint that eventually Mathew felt that he had rather used Stephens for his own ends; in one of his rather cringing letters to Milnes (15 Aug 1848) [8] he entreats Milnes to send a complimentary copy of his *Biography of Keats* to Stephens. Interestingly he also entreats Milnes to send a copy to Miss Severn of Bolt Court (Fleet Street) as she had introduced him to Stephens. Miss Emma Severn was the sister of Charles Severn who was a contemporary of Keats, Stephens and Mackereth during their student days. She seems not to have been related to Joseph Severn, who painted portraits of Keats and who accompanied him on his terminal visit to Rome.

Beyond Medical Studies

In March 1817, free of medical commitments, Keats went to live with his brothers in Well Walk adjoining Hampstead Heath. Here he was in more relaxed, rural surroundings, closer to his friends both literary and political, but not far from London's theatres and museums. Here he could devote himself to creative poetry and the social network that nurtured it. With the help of solitary or semi-solitary visits to the Isle of Wight, Oxford and Stratford-upon-Avon he completed his first long epic poem, *Endymion.* But shortly after his return from Oxford in October, as Tom was visibly ailing with what would prove to be tuberculosis, he himself was briefly ill with a condition that was improved or cured with " *...a little mercury...* " which "... *corrected the Poison and improved my Health...*".

Much effort has been put into either diagnosing this illness or dismissing it. Mercury was prescribed almost exclusively for venereal diseases at that date. A likely opinion advocated by Gittings[1] is that he had contracted gonorrhoea during his visit to Oxford, a condition that was relatively common among young men. It was less life-threatening than syphilis and also attracted less social disapprobation. Contemporary medical opinion had no knowledge of the bacterial origin of either of these diseases and, moreover, believed gonorrhoea to be an early stage of syphilis; it recommended as treatment small doses of mercury for gonorrhoea and larger doses for syphilis. Keats must have been aware of this treatment from his student days but it was also recommended by Dr Solomon Sawrey who was now attending both Tom and himself and who had previously written a treatise on *An Inquiry into Some of the Effects of the Venereal Poison* (1802)[1].

Heavier doses of mercury were prescribed for Keats about a year later. He still lived in Well Walk and was still nursing the deteriorating Tom. But he had lately returned from his walking expedition in Scotland with the indefatigable and adventurous Charles Brown, a neighbour from Hampstead's Wentworth Place. This expedition of about a month had encountered some of the anticipated wonders, such as the hills and waterfalls around Grasmere, the geological architecture of Fingal's Cave and the terrifying isolation of the summit of Ben Nevis in mist. Even if it also provided depressing impressions of the deprived poverty of some rural areas, there was plenty to enrich the poetic imagination and to guide Keats' endless self-analysis. But the cost of the expedition was the physical exertion and deprivations that the travellers endured. They walked in all about 600 miles [4] perhaps the most exhausting being the 37 miles across the bogs and moors of Mull in bad weather and having to sleep in wet clothes on the earth floors of peasants' cottages.

The robust Brown was relatively unaffected, but Keats lost weight, developed a severe cold with a badly ulcerated throat [1], and was advised by a doctor in Inverness to return home by boat. Although he seems to have recovered his spirits on the return voyage and so arrived in Hampstead threadbare but lively, he was soon back to his nursing duties with the terminally ill Tom. But between August and September he was dosing himself with mercury sufficient to produce recognised symptoms. Gittings concludes that he was taking it, on Sawtry's advice, in case the throat condition was a syphilitic ulcer. This proved not to be the case, but was nevertheless worrying. Mercury was prescribed only reluctantly, and was thought to be particularly dangerous to tubercular patients. Whether or not the mercury predisposed Keats to contract tuberculosis from Tom, it is likely that Keats himself believed it did [1].

As Tom lay dying, which occurred on 1 December (Wells [4] mistakes this for 18th), Keats had also to endure the reviews of his early poems and *Endymion* in *Blackwood's Magazine*. These were clever, vicious, biting and politically motivated. They came from a very conservative background, identified Keats with the radical attitudes of Hunt and his friends and mocked him for his humbler "cockney" background and his medical training. *"... so back to the shop, Mr John, back to the plasters, pills, and ointment boxes."* His robust friend, the critic William Hazlitt, was also personally attacked in the same issue of *Blackwood's*, but so furiously sued the editors that they settled with him out of Court [1]. Hazlitt referred to the critical thrust from *Blackwood's* that struck Keats *"...the shaft was spite, venal, vulgar, venomous..."* . Along with Shelley he was of the opinion that this criticism, acting on the sensitive and susceptible Keats, somehow

41

induced physical damage to his lungs. Many of those who knew him well, including brother George, Fanny Brawne and Cowden Clarke, were also convinced that the criticisms were in some way directly responsible for his early death. Many biographers have commented on what Wells [4] calls the Keats legend: " *Indeed there is a romantic appeal in the story of the talented, sensitive young poet who droops and dies like a tender plant, under the withering blasts of unfriendly criticism.*"

Later biographers, including Wells [4] who writes from a medical perspective, have indeed acknowledged that these bitter, highly personal and anonymous attacks, coming at a time when his personal circumstances were distressing, hurt Keats very much indeed; they affected his reputation among the reading public and so greatly diminished sales of his books. But the biographers also emphasise his resilience and self-awareness and argue that they never really undermined his belief, as he expressed it to George: " *I think I shall be among the English poets after my death*" [4]. The best of Keats was yet to come. Wells writes *"It is remarkable nevertheless, that it was during this time of trouble and misfortune – the unfriendly criticism, the illness and loss of his brother, depleted finances, worsening health, a hopeless love affair – that he produced his greatest poetry. During a period extending from the fall of 1818 to the fall 1819, Keats... plunged into the most amazingly creative year that any English poet has ever achieved. Gittings calls it the "Living Year".*

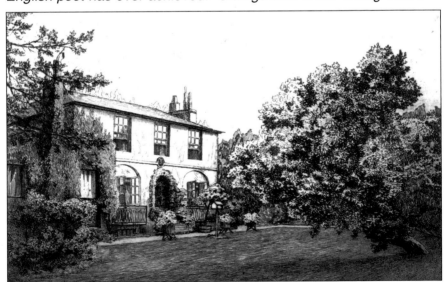

(fig 16)   KEATS HOUSE, HAMPSTEAD in 1907
By this date, the two semi-detached houses of Wentworth Place had been merged into one, Lawn Bank.
(Keats House Hampstead, London)

Soon after Tom's death, Keats went to live as a paying guest with his friend Charles Brown in Wentworth Place at the edge of Hampstead Heath. It was half of the substantial villa that now forms the commemorative Keats House. He stayed here with Brown for some seventeen months, so that the house witnessed the writing of many of his odes, the lung haemorrhage that foretold his fate and, poignantly, the near presence of Fanny Brawne, the object of his obsessive love, whose widowed mother brought her family to live in the adjoining half of the house in April, 1819. He had met Fanny at a social occasion probably in November just before Tom's death. The occasion is obscure, but there must have been initial frissons and it is argued [1] that it is to the 18-year-old Fanny that the sonnet *Bright Star!* was addressed. A teasing, flirtatious courtship developed over the period of Keats' grieving, possibly to his great benefit.

Fanny (Frances) was the eldest child of a youngish widow, also Frances Brawne, whose husband had earlier died of tuberculosis leaving her with three children and a small but adequate pension. As the courtship developed and Fanny became increasingly the object of Keats' affections and passion, her presence next door presented him with extra problems. His attentions and infatuation with Fanny would be visible to his friends and to Fanny's mother. He had no money for marital ambitions and no financial expectation; his health was far from good and not improving; and he must have wondered whether marriage was compatible with his poetic aspirations. The relationship, which was not approved of by Brown and some other friends, seemed increasingly doomed. In spite of these objections and its built-in frustrations and jealousies, the infatuation strengthened and by the end of 1819 the couple were formally engaged. To simplify a complex relationship, one could say that *Bright Star!* was now *La Belle Dame sans Merci.* For the rest of his life, Keats was, in this matter, *in thrall.*

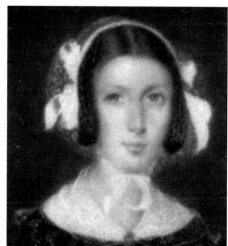

(fig 17)   FANNY BRAWNE (1800-1865)
Her genuine love for Keats was not appreciated until her letters to Keats' sister Fanny were published in 1937 (Keats House)

The last years of Keats' life, from 1819 to his death in Rome on 23 February 1821, were constrained by complex often insoluble problems. The biographies quoted have examined at length how in spite of these, in 1819 he created enduring poetry including many of his odes. They examine how far the poetry was evoked and influenced by these problems and also by Keats' endless struggles to understand the philosophical basis of human understanding and experience. Keats House evokes only some of the external factors that triggered this poetic outburst. The relatively secluded garden makes it easy to imagine how the nightingale's song could evoke a poetic reverie, but not the elaborate, melancholic imagery of Keats' ode. But a bedroom in the house makes it easy to imagine how Brown saw Keats, distressed, cold and feverish from a long journey on the top of a coach, examining by candle-light the blood he had just coughed from his lungs, and concluding " ...*it is arterial blood. I cannot be deceived in that colour; That drop of blood is my death warrant; I must die* ..." [1,2,4]

This haemorrhage was in February 1820, just over a year after the death of Tom. Biographers including the medical Wells [4] emphasise the certainty of Keats' diagnosis which was based on his medical training and also on his family experiences. What perplexes the biographers are the diagnoses produced by his doctors and the treatments that they prescribed. Local doctors were quickly in attendance both to bleed him and put him onto a very restricted diet. This, of course, produced no improvement and so Dr Robert Bree of Hanover Square, London, an eminent specialist in disordered respiration and a physician to royalty, was consulted. Wells [4] tries to reconstruct the doctor's knowledge and the degree to which he would have examined his patient physically; in 1820, it must be recalled, not only was the bacterial nature of consumption not recognised (*Mycobacterium tuberculosis*; Robert Koch, 1884 [10]), but even auscultation of the chest with a primitive stethoscope almost unknown. Dr Bree diagnosed excessive nervous irritability and anxiety and suggested that he avoided poetry and studied mathematics instead; to Keats' relief however he was taken off his starvation diet and allowed to eat meat and drink light wine.

The medical advice Keats received following a second haemorrhage in June was no better. By now he was lodging in Kentish Town, for Brown, as was his habit, had rented his house for the summer and gone on a walking tour in Scotland. Leigh Hunt had realised that Keats was now in some distress and had found him inexpensive lodgings at Wesleyan Place near to his own house. Here he was able to revise some of his poetry for publication but was tormented by separation from Fanny and furiously jealous to learn of her few social excursions. Following his haemorrhage he was attended by Dr George Darling who bled him, while Dr William Lambe, called in as an eminent consultant, further restricted his diet and made it vegetarian. The disease and the doctors' treatment of it reduced Keats to a pathetic, wasted condition. There seemed no hope of his surviving the English winter and he was recommended, or rather ordered to Italy, a warmer climate, immediately.

The slow boat journey to Italy in an inadequate brig, sharing its one overcrowded cabin with many others, including a young lady who was also consumptive, and with delays due to bad weather on the English coast and a quarantine period in the harbour at Naples, is the stuff of nightmares and has passed into literary legend. There were a few rays of sunshine before this storm. His second book of poems, including *The Eve of St Agnes, Lamia*, and major Odes, was published and well received. Moreover, he had been accepted by Mrs Brawne into her household to be nursed by herself and Fanny for his last four weeks in England. Mrs Brawne did not have much choice in this arrangement. Ill, tearful and confused he had left Hunt's house following a minor mishap, and walked and crawled to the house in Well Walk where Tom had died and then on to the Brawne doorstep in Wentworth Place. His state was such that Mrs Brawne had to abandon discretion and take him in.

Almost in extremis he was now in the place where he would have wished to be, and with Fanny. But the voyage to Italy could not be avoided. Organised and mostly paid for by his friends, the journey started from Hampstead on 13 September. The pressing question as to who was to accompany him on his odyssey was resolved when Joseph Severn, the painter, volunteered. The ability of Keats to attract an extraordinary degree of love and attention from his friends has been well described. Severn proved to be one such friend. Not only did he endure the journey and settle Keats into lodgings in the Piazza di Spagna in Rome, he was with him on 23 February 1821 when, late in the evening, he died.

Assuming that Keats had contracted consumption while nursing Tom in the confined rooms in Well Walk, the course of the disease had lasted about 27 months. It is difficult not to compare this with the similar time (30 months) that Stephens' first wife, Hannah, lived after her marriage in September 1829 [5] and to consider the poignant possibility that she was already infected with the tubercle bacillus at the time of her marriage.

References: John Keats

1   Gittings, R. (1971) *John Keats.* Penguin Books Ltd, Harmondworth, Middlesex.

2   Motion, A. (1997) *Keats.* Farrar, Straus and Giroux, New York.

3   Colvin, S.   (1917)   *John Keats.* Macmillan and Co. Ltd, London.

4   Wells, W.A. (1959)   *A Doctor's Life of John Keats.* Vantage Press Inc., New York.

5   Pierpoint, W.S. (This script) *Unparallel Lives... Part 1. Henry Stephens.*

6   Renier, H.   (2006)   *Lambeth Past.* Historical Publications, London.

7   South, J.F. (1884)   *Memorials* (Ed. C.L. Feltoe), John Murray, Albemarle Street, London.

8   Rollins, H.E. (1948) Ed. *The Keats Circle.* Vol. 2. Harvard University Press, Cambridge, Mass, USA.

9   Barnard, J. (2007) Ed. *John Keats. Selected Poems.* Penguin Books, London.

10 Bigger, J.B. (1949) *Handbook of Bacteriology.* Bailliere, Tindall and Cox, London.

GEORGE WILSON MACKERETH (1793-1869)

A PERSISTENT PRACTITIONER

George Wilson Mackereth was born in March 1793 in the now "lost" village of Owthorne in the East Riding of Yorkshire, and baptised, without his middle name, in the Parish church of St Peter on the 10th [1]. His father, "John Mackereth, Clerk..." was curate to the parish, having been appointed around 1787. In 1811 John was presented with the living as vicar [2]. However, as the old parish church, endangered by disrepair and by coastal erosion, was being dismantled, his responsibilities were transferred to the new (1801) church at nearby Rimswell and later probably extended to the non-residential curacy in Ottringham . The County History [3] records that a John Mackereth was appointed curate here in 1811 and that he was aided by his son Miles, who later succeeded him as curate then vicar (1848-1881).

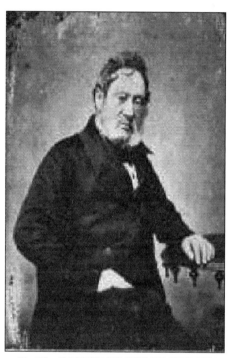

(fig 18)   GEORGE WILSON MACKERETH
in later life
Houghton Library, Harvard University,
MS Keats 10 (27)

Background and Apprenticeship
We assume that these two John Mackereths, both vicars, are the same man, so that Miles is George Mackereth's brother.   John probably settled in Ottringham eventually, for the census of the village in 1841 lists an 80-year-old John Mackereth living there with Ann, presumably his wife, age 75 years.   Miles also settled in Ottringham until he retired to Patrington where he died (1881);   the Ottringham census of 1861 finds him entertaining a visitor, Arthur A. Mackereth, a mariner aged 31, who is very likely to be his nephew, Arthur Augustus, the second son of brother George Wilson.

John's living at Owthorne may have been rewarding enough to contribute eventually to his son's medical training, but it could not have been without its anxieties. Ancient Owthorne was then an exposed village standing directly on a bluff overlooking the North Sea. The boulder clay on which it was built suffered much from *"...the encroachments of the sea, which are averaged at from 1-2½ yards annually along the coast..."*. Guidebooks list over 20 villages and a priory on a short stretch of coast north from Spurn Head which have been lost to the sea since medieval times. Fields and dwellings in Owthorne were gradually eroded and, with permission, the chancel of the church was dismantled in 1793 followed by much of the rest of it in 1799 [3]. The *coup de grace* came following a very high spring tide on the night of Friday February 24, 1816 [4]; this undercut the tower and what remained of the church and churchyard and they fell on Saturday afternoon *"...into the bosom of the ocean ..."*. The old vicarage was adjacent to the church but managed to survive until 1846 when, as one of the last houses in the village, it too was taken by the sea. But as it was said to have been uninhabitable in 1764, and its inland replacement on the Hull road was not built until 1847, it is not clear which was the family home of the youthful George Mackereth, and his siblings including Elisabeth (b.1796)[1] and probably Miles (ca.1804-1881).

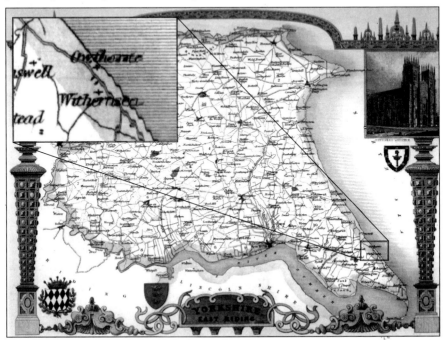

(fig 19)   THE EAST RIDING OF YORKSHIRE c.1830.
Part of map by Thomas Moule.

It is unclear from where young Mackereth got the impulse to become a doctor or why he did not receive his initial training in Hull or a neighbouring village. But his latter registration with the Society of Apothecaries of London indicates that he served his five-year apprenticeship south of the Humber with a "Thomas Copeland" of Winterton (Lincs). This is almost certainly Thomas Coopland, surgeon (1787-1826) who, along with two sons, is buried in Winterton parish church and commemorated there by a wall-plaque [5]. But by 1815 Mackereth had left these remote, rural villages, possibly by boat, and was established in overcrowded, dirty, metropolitan Southwark.

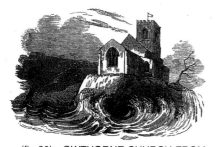

(fig 20) OWTHORNE CHURCH FROM THE SEA, 1806
The History and Antiquities of Holderness by G Poulson 1841
(British Library Board RB, 31.c.304)

Medical Studies in London

He registered as a 12-month pupil at Guy's and St Thomas' Hospitals on October 16, having paid his office fees of £1.2.0 on the 4th. Hospital archives [6] record his presence and payment of fees, and they also confirm his reluctance to use his middle name and that he had been apprenticed to Dr Coopland. He must have met Stephens early in his stay and they quickly established themselves in the house of Mr Markham, the tallow-chandler, at 28 St Thomas Street, possibly sharing a sitting room with another student [7]. This meeting led to a life-long friendship between Mackereth and Stephens. But friendship between Mackereth and Keats, who came to share their sitting room in December, was less enduring.

Mackereth's activities over the next 16 or so months must have resembled those of Keats and Stephens with both of whom he was a constant companion. They would have included the long hours of lectures and practical work, walking the wards and witnessing their misery and distress, and attending the crowded, terrifying operating theatre. They would also have included such extramural student delights as cards, claret, and theatres; it is easy to imagine that excursions across the busy Thames into the City and beyond caused wonder and excitement in the young countryman, but it is clear that they never weakened his affection for the quieter Yorkshire coastlands.

There are but passing references to Mackereth in the authoritative biographies of Keats by Colvin, Gittings and Motion, and the most recent one [8] concludes that after Mackereth gained his LSA at the second attempt, he entirely disappeared from Keats' life. His seal and his autograph were eventually presented by one of his sons to the Keats Collection at Harvard [9], but he seems not to have recorded his memories of the young poet. It can safely be assumed that he shared Stephens' somewhat suspicious and resentful attitude towards Keats, an assumption supported by the one anecdote specifically involving him that survives [8].

Both Mackereth and Keats resolved to undergo their LSA examination in July 1816 although Stephens, unsure of his ability in Latin, decided to postpone his own ordeal. Both candidates were examined orally, probably for an hour or two, at the Apothecaries Hall in Blackfriars Lane, just north of the river, on 25 July; but whereas Keats was successful, Mackereth, examined by the chairman of the panel, was rejected. He carried this gloomy news back to his lodgings, and is supposed to have had a conversation with Stephens that stirred up the surprise and resentment at Keats' success that was later articulated by Stephens when he himself was rejected by the examiners on August 22. The source of this well-quoted incident is not clear. It is not specifically mentioned in Stephens' reminiscences [10].

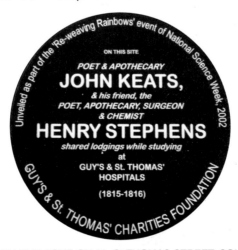

(fig 21)   BLUE PLAQUE ON 28, St THOMAS STREET, SOUTHWARK

It is possible, but not recorded, that Mackereth was present in the lodgings in St Thomas Street on the warm, muggy, summer day in 1816 when the local "resurrection men" under the leadership of the formidable Ben Crouch deposited a corpse [11]. This was to assist the anatomical studies of the former resident, George Cooper, who was now in practice at Brentford. Markham had undertaken to wax the body for its dispatch to Brentford by the Thames and had enlisted the help of his student lodgers. Their embalming efforts were, no doubt, adequate for the occasion, but did not prevent the corpse, in a hamper, from becoming an odorously unpleasant fellow-passenger to others on the boat. The incident, parenthetically, suggests why Markham located his tallow-chandler business close to the hospitals.

> The mode in which the exhumation was performed by the adepts was not, as might have been supposed, by digging out the newly-filled earth from the not very deep grave, and exposing the coffin lid, and, after removing, to take out the corpse, but they found it most convenient to dig down at the head of the grave, knock in the end of the coffin, and drag the body out. It was then disrobed from the shroud, which was most carefully put back into the coffin, to avoid committing a felony, the disturbance of the grave and taking the corpse being merely a misdemeanour. The subject was then doubled up into the smallest possible compass, and either thrust into a coarse sack or an orange basket—if in season—and laid aside till as many graves as were convenient had been despoiled.

(fig 22)   THE RESURRECTION MEN
Description of the methods used by the "resurrection men" to rob graves,
John Flint South's "Memorials" (ref 6, p.28).

After the winter (1816) course of surgery with Sir Astley Cooper, Mackereth took the examination with the Corporation of Surgeons on 7 March (1817) and was admitted as an MRCS. Stephens had preceded him on 7 February along with fellow-student Henry Newmarch, a light-hearted friend of the Keats family who had often pleased Stephens and Mackereth by pricking some of the poetic pretensions of Keats. Keats himself never finished the surgery course nor took the examination. Under the literary spell of Leigh Hunt and his circle and having seen his poetry in print, he had taken his brave and celebrated decision to forsake medicine and devote himself to poetry.

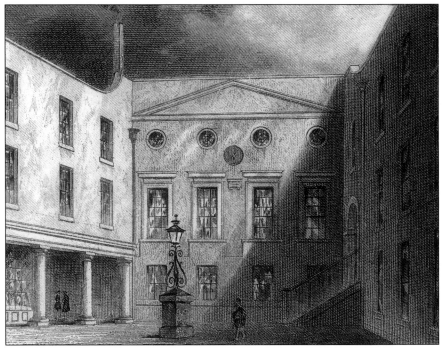

*(fig 23)   Courtyard Entrance to APOTHECARIES HALL, Blackfriars Lane
(Worshipful Society of Apothecaries of London)*

But before Mackereth and Stephens could be qualified to set up independent practices they had to resit the LSA examinations that they had failed some months earlier. They both took some trouble revising Latin although there is no evidence that Mackereth, unlike Stephens, visited Keats in his lodgings in Cheapside to do so; he was not present at the birth of the first line of *Endymion*. Both were examined, successfully, on 1 March 1817. Both their licences were provincial, indicating that they could only practise "in the country", that is anywhere in England and Wales outside a ten-mile radius of London.   These were not lesser qualifications, but they required a smaller registration fee of £6 instead of £10. They suggest that both men intended to take their talents back into the countryside.

Mackereth back in Yorkshire

George Mackereth, albeit without his characteristic middle name, is listed in the comprehensive directories of medical men of Hull and of the East Riding of Yorkshire compiled by Dr and Mrs Bickford [12,13]. He must have moved directly back to the East Riding and he is listed as being in practice in the village of Preston a few miles east of Hull between 1819-1822 [12]. Half of his practising life was spent in small towns in the low, undulating and well-watered plain of Holderness, principally Keyingham, although between 1837 and 1858 he lived more urbanely in Hull. As the towns and villages were small and not far removed from each other his practice must have extended to cover a group of them as well as the isolated farmsteads between. His horse must have been familiar with the muddy country roads and farm tracks at all times of the day and in all weathers. He may have attended wealthier patients in Hull and the larger country houses, but as parish records show he also attended the impoverished sick in Burton Pidsea at the request of the *"...overseers of the poor..."* [13].

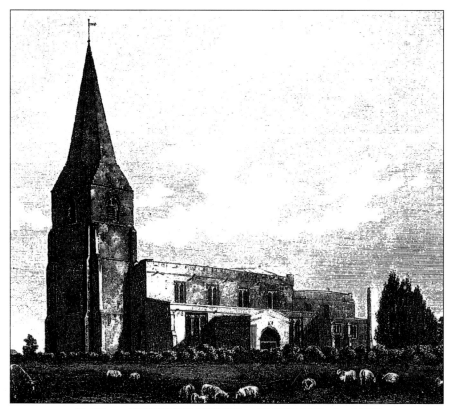

(fig 24)   KEYINGHAM CHURCH,   HOLDERNESS, about 1830
The History and Antiquities of Holderness by G Poulson 1841
(British Library Board RB,31.c.304)

In 1824 he married Margaret Sarah Brown (1804-1891), a farmer's daughter from the hamlet of Ganstead, in the church at Swine. Soon afterwards they may have settled nearer Keyingham, for the first seven of their nine children, born between 1827 (John Frederick) and 1839 (Alethea) are all either born [1] or baptised [13] there. The two further daughters were born in Hull; Margaret Agnes in 1841 and

Mary Fanny in 1843 or 4. Margaret Agnes was too late to be included in the first census returns of 1841 which reveal that the family then lived in Paradise Row in the Hull parish of Holy Trinity. This accommodation may have been relatively modest as their neighbours were working folk including farm labourers; it may also have been rather crowded with six children in the house.

The family seems to have avoided the census of 1851, when they lived in the more prominent Prospect Street. By 1861 they had moved back to Keyingham to Church Lane House, but by then only the four youngest girls, Sarah, Alethea, Margaret Agnes and Mary Fanny, still lived with their parents. Their neighbours included a Veterinary Surgeon but again were mostly rural working people. The censuses give no evidence that the Mackereths employed resident servants.

George's practice clearly extended beyond the boundaries of the village of Keyingham. His attendance on the poor of Burton Pidsea, about five miles distant, has already been mentioned. In 1859 he acted for the Admiralty as both surgeon and agent, in the small naval settlements of Paull, Easington and Holmpton scattered some 6-11 miles away on the coast or the Humber estuary [14]. But his regional activities extended also to commercial interests. While still in Hull (1847) he was, as the Bickfords discovered [2], party to the sale of the leasehold of the manor of Ottringham *"All that excellent and commodious messuage or dwelling house, with the large School room, stable, hay chamber and other conveniences adjoining thereto. Also that excellent orchard...and close of valuable pasture land, amounting to about 4 acres 3 roods; the above premises all adjoining, situate on the west side of the High Road from Ottringham to Halsham. Also those four excellent and substantially built tenements, each containing two "low" rooms, two chambers, a dairy or pantry and other conveniences...with four gardens adjoining."*

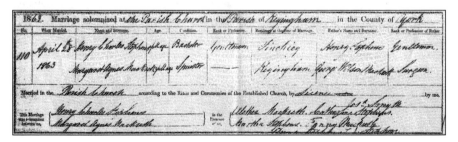

(fig 25)   REGISTRATION OF MARRIAGE between Stephens' son Henry Charles and Mackereth's daughter Margaret Agnes 1863.

The County Archives contain other Mackereth indentures of this period (1848 and 1852) [2]. Such business activities continued at Keyingham and an indenture dated 1860 is interesting in that it involves Samuel Josiah Stephens of Charlotte Street, Marylebone, Middlesex, who was the younger, entrepreneurial brother of Henry Stephens: moreover his signature is witnessed by his clerk Henry John Stephens who was almost certainly the nephew of both Samuel and Henry Stephens, the son of their deceased elder brother John (1795-1846). This business visit of the brother and nephew of Henry Stephens indicates that the close, continuous connection between Mackereth and Stephens must have extended to their families as well.

This close connection became closer in 1863 when Mackereth's 21-year-old daughter, Margaret Agnes, married Henry Charles (22), the eldest child of Henry Stephens. Henry Charles had been educated in Paris and University College School in London and had joined the family business making good-quality inks and woodstains. He continued his studies of both chemistry and business management and took over management of this successful business when his father died in 1864 [15]. The wedding took place in Keyingham on April 28, in the Parish Church. Stephens' daughter Martha Walsh later (1925)[16] remembered the occasion …

> *"The wedding took place at Keyingham, near Hull, where Mackreth was then in practice and very popular. We all went down to be present, also Uncle [Samuel] Josiah and aunt Mary Anne, my father (in good health and spirits) with my mother. Everything went off splendidly."*

It is interesting that on signing the marriage certificate, Mackereth describes himself as a *Surgeon*; Stephens, his medical days now past, describes himself as a *Gentleman*. It is even more interesting that the announcement of the wedding in *The Times* (2 May, 1863), records that the service was principally conducted by the *"... Rev. Miles Mackreth, uncle of the bride..."*. Miles, then the vicar at nearby Ottringham, is clearly brother to George Wilson Mackereth.

(fig 26)   MARGARET AGNES STEPHENS
about 1866
(The Stephens Collection)

The married couple went to live at Grove House in Finchley. Ten years later (1874) Henry Charles and Agnes purchased nearby Avenue House with its adjacent land, developing both house and gardens extensively. Henry proved to be a successful and energetic business man, acquiring the sobriquet "Inky Stephens" as the business expanded. He went into politics both local and national, serving three terms as a Conservative M.P. for the Hornsey Division of Middlesex before retiring in 1900 on a matter of principle. In addition he developed a large country estate of about 5,000 acres at Cholderton, on the Hampshire/Wiltshire border, where he introduced up-to-the-minute methods of farm management, animal breeding and water extraction [15]. Avenue House was eventually (1918) bequeathed by Stephens to the people of Finchley; although it and its garden have been adapted to municipal uses, it still has a small museum and Collection devoted to the history of the Stephens family. Henry Stephens did not long survive his son's marriage. He died eighteen months later (September, 1864) at Farringdon Street Station while returning from a business trip to London [16].

It is possible that Mackereth attended his friend's funeral in Finchley, for he survived another five years. He was still listed in Medical Directories until 1870. But in 1867 he shortened his name to Mackreth, presumably to match the spelling preferred by his medical son, John Frederick, so that their names appeared juxtaposed in the Medical Directories. Sometime in the next two years he seems to have retired and he and his wife moved from Keyingham to Scarborough. By 1869 the directories list him as address unknown, but John Frederick is now in Keyingham and has presumably taken over his father's practice.

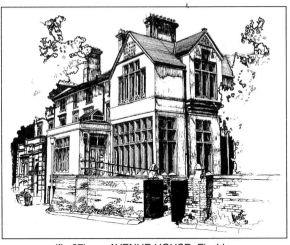

(fig 27)   AVENUE HOUSE Finchley,
The home of Henry & Margaret Stephens
(The Stephens Collection)

Mackereth died, aged 75, in his house Inkerman Villa, Scarborough, after a series of apoplectic attacks, in March 1869. His death was reported by John Frederick (1828-1900), who, incidentally, had been trained at Erlangen, Bavaria (MD), Edinburgh (LRCP) as well as Guy's & St Thomas' (MRCS). The funeral took place on 8 March in the church at Hedon in Holderness, about five miles east of Keyingham [2]. There seems to be no known memorial stone to mark his grave as they do for his two medical colleagues, Stephens and Keats. An eroded stone memorial to George Wilson Mackereth in St Augustine's churchyard in Hedon marks the grave of someone else (1820-1846), possibly a relative, of the same name [2].

By 1869 the posthumous reputation of John Keats had grown enormously [17]. Sometime after Mackereth's death, John Frederick was visited either by F.H. Day, an eccentric American collector of Keatsiana, or by his agent, and gave him Mackereth's seal and autograph [10]. These could not be located, as Rollins [10] suggested, in the catalogue of the Keats collection at Harvard. The catalogue search, however, unexpectedly revealed the pencil drawing of the young Mackereth (cover and Fig 28) and the photograph of him in later life (Fig 18); the drawing is listed as having come from Day and is, tentatively and surprisingly, attributed to Keats' devoted friend, Joseph Severn.

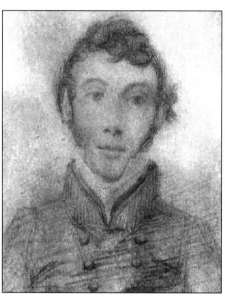

(fig 28) Sketch of George MACKERETH Attributed tentatively to Joseph Severn by F.H. Day

Mackereth's name was kept alive for some time when a son was born to John Frederick in Gilling, just north of Richmond, in 1859 and was christened John Frederick George Wilson Mackereth [1]. This grandson seems not to have followed in the medical footsteps of his father and grandfather. The 1901 census finds him *"living on own means"* in what may have been his father's house in Keyingham; he had two servants and a *"boarder"* who was a *"medical practitioner Surg"*. Then he and his grandiloquent name disappear from the records.

Margaret, wife of George Wilson Mackereth, died aged 85 in Scarborough in 1891. She did not share her husband's grave, but was buried in nearby Hutton Buscel. [12]

References: George Wilson Mackereth

1   Names and dates have been obtained on-line using computer searches of IGI data, censuses and BDM records obtained via *Family History* or *Ancestry* sources.

2   Mrs M. Bickford. Personal communication.

3   Victoria History of the Counties of England: East Riding of Yorkshire, vol V (1984). Institute of Historical Research.

4   *Hull Advertiser.* 24th Feb. 1816.

5   Mr S. Stubbins. Personal communication.

6   Records in Archival Library of King's College, Strand, London.

7   Pierpoint, W.S. (This script) *Unparallel Lives... Part 1. Henry Stephens.*

8   Motion, A. (1997) *Keats.* Faber & Faber, London.

9   Rollins, H.E. (1948) Ed. *The Keats Circle*, Vol. 2, p. 207 footnote. Harvard University Press, Cambridge, Mass, USA.

10 Rollins, H.E. (1948) Ed. *The Keats Circle*, Vol. 2, pp. 206-214. Harvard University Press, Cambridge, Mass. USA.

11 Gittings, R. (1971) *John Keats.* Penguin Books, London.

12 Bickford, J.A.R, Bickford, M.E. (2007). *East Riding Medical Men.* East Yorkshire Family History Society.

13 Bickford, J.A.R, Bickford M.E. (1983) *The Medical Profession in Hull.* Kingston upon Hull City Council Publication.

14 Medical Directories. In the collection of The Wellcome Library, Euston Road, London.

15 Musgrove, P. (1984) *Henry C. Stephens.* London, The Finchley Society.

16 Walsh, M. (1925) *The Life of Henry Stephens.* The Stephens Collection, London.

17 Plumly, S, (2008) *Posthumous Keats.* W.W. Norton, New York and London.

ENVOY

" ...He [Keats] died as I have since understood at Rome at the age
of 25, and out of 6 Medical Students who at that time associated
together, myself & another only are left, but the world goes on, other
young men with similar feelings and similar associations rise upon the
Stage, & play their parts & go off as others have done before, & their
loss though felt in their own circle is not much known beyond it..."

Henry Stephens
(Letter to G.F. Mathew, March 1847)

ACKNOWLEDGEMENTS

I gratefully acknowledge the help, advice and encouragement that has been given to me by Mrs and the late Dr J.A.R. Bickford of Kirk Ella, Hull. Not only were their published works on medical men of the East Riding very useful, but they have made freely available to me unpublished researches and have helped to check my own findings and put them in perspective. My wife Maureen has been very helpful in many expected and unexpected ways. It was her sharp eyes that spotted the records of Stephens' first marriage in seemingly interminable rolls of microfilm in the London Metropolitan Archives. The sharp eyes and professional judgement of Mr Peter Marsh and Mr Stewart Wild, both of The Stephens Collection, Avenue House, Finchley, made the manuscript presentable.

I have received kind and courteous help from the staff of London Metropolitan Archives (Northampton Road, London), Hertfordshire Archives and Local Studies (Hertford), The Archive Room at King's College Library (Strand, London), The Wellcome Library for the History of Medicine (Euston Road, London), The Stephens Collection (Avenue House, Finchley), Keats House (Mr K. Page; Hampstead, London), The Pen Room (Hockley, Birmingham), The Guildhall Library (Aldermanbury, London), the Libraries of The Apothecaries Society of London (Black Friars Lane), the Royal College of Surgeons (Lincoln's Inn Fields, London), the Archive Manager of the East Riding Council, at Beverley (Mr Ian Mason), the Newspaper section of the British Library in Colindale (N. London), and the Houghton Library, Harvard University (Heather Cole).

It is difficult to list all those who have provided specialist or local information and encouragement. Mr S. Stubbins of Winterton located the memorial plaque to Dr Coopland, formerly of that town. M/s T. Humphrey (Beccles; Essex) gave me information on printing factories in Southwark, Drs Geoff. Bateman (Harpenden, Herts), D.H. Leaback (Radlett, Herts) and Dr Denis Gibbs (Appleford, Oxon) guided me, mentally, around Holderness, Southwark and the History of Medicine respectively. I thank them all.

Every reasonable effort has been made to trace copyright holders of material reproduced in this booklet, but if any have been inadvertently overlooked, the author and publishers apologise sincerely.

William S. Pierpoint, August 2010

Index

A

Abbey, Richard (Keats' guardian) .. 33, 38
Apothecary Act (1815) 34
Apothecaries Hall 50, 52
The Asclepiad 6, 28
Avenue House, Finchley 27, 56

B

Biography of Keats 40, 58
Blackwood's magazine 41
Blue plaque 3
Brawne, Fanny 43
Brawne, Frances 43, 45
Bree, Dr Robert 44
Brentford 5, 51
Bright Star! 43
Broad Street, Soho 16, 19
Brown, Charles 11, 31, 41, 44
Brown, Margaret Sarah 53
Bull Inn, Redbourn 1, 9, 10, 39
Burton Pidsea, East Yorks 53, 54
Byron 13

C

Calloway, Thomas 15
Charlotte Street 12, 55
Cholderton, Wilts 56
Cholera 12, 15-19
Clarke, Charles Cowden ....
.... 4, 32, 32, 34, 35, 37
Clarke, John 32
Clarke's school 32, 33, 34
Coastal erosion, East Yorks 48
Consumption *see* Tuberculosis
Cooper, Sir Astley 4, 9, 10, 35, 51
Cooper, Bransby 13
Cooper, George 3, 5, 35, 36, 50
Coopland, Thomas 49
Cowper, William 11

D

Darling, Dr George 44

E

Edmonton, London 33
Endymion 6, 7, 40, 41
Enfield, Middx 32
Excursion into the North
  Henry Stephens 11, 28
  John Keats 11, 41

F

Faraday, Michael 25
Farringdon Street station 26, 27, 56
Finchley 21, 24, 25, 26, 55, 56
The Finchley Society 25

G

Gadebridge 10
Gorhambury estate 9, 10
Grove House, Finchley 21, 24, 56
Guy's Hospital 2, 20, 34, 35, 56

H

Hammond, Thomas 33, 34
Hampstead 40-43
Harvard University 50, 57
Hazlitt, William 38, 39, 41
Hedon, East Yorks 57
Hernia treatment 10, 13, 14, 15, 28
Hunt, Leigh 5, 6, 37, 38, 44, 51
Hyperion 11

I

Ink, manufacturing 20-22, 24

J

Jennings, John 31, 32
Johnson, James 17

K

Keats

Edward (1801-02) 31
Fanny (Frances Mary b.1803) 32
Frances (1775-1810) 31, 33
George (b.1797) 9, 11, 38
Georgiana 9, 11, 39
John (1795-1821)
.... 4, 7, 31, 33, 36, 43-44, death 45, 49
Thomas (1773-1804) 31, 32
Tom (1799-1818) 31, 40, 41
Keats' poems and odes 45
Keyingham, East Yorks 26, 52, 55, 56
Koch, Robert 16, 17, 44

L

Lamb, Charles 38, 39
Lambe, Dr William 44
Liverpool 11, 39

M

Mackereth

Ann (b.1766) 47
Arthur (b.1830) 47
Elisabeth (b.1796) 48
George Wilson (1793-1869)
.... 3, 6, 26, 31, death 56, 57
John (b.1761) 47
John Frederick (1828-1900) 56, 57
Margaret, née Brown (1804-91) 57
Margaret Agnes (b.1841) 26, 53
Miles (c.1804-81) 47, 48, 55
Marcet, Alexander 4, 20

Markham (tallow-chandler) 3, 5, 36, 49, 51
Markyate, Herts 1, 34
Mathew, George Felton 7, 37, 39, 40
Mechanics' Magazine 23
Medical Society of London 13, 29
Metropolitan Railway 26
Milnes, Richard Monkton
  (Lord Houghton) 6, 40
Monkhouse, Thomas 39
Motion, Andrew 8, 28, 33, 46
Musgrove, Paddy 21, 29

N

Nash, Ebenezer 21, 22
Newmarch, Henry 51

O

Ottringham, East Yorks 47, 54, 55
Owen, Richard 8
Owthorne, East Yorks 47, 48

P

Patents 22, 28
Poems by Keats 45
Piazza di Spagna, Rome 45
Preston, East Yorks 52

R

Rawlings, William 32
Redbourn .... 1 ,9, 28, 39
Reilly (O'Reilly) 19
Renier, Hannah 35
Resurrectionists 5, 51
Richardson, Sir Benjamin 6, 11, 25, 28
Royal College of Surgeons 2
Royal Institution 25

S

St Botolph's Without 31
St Thomas' Hospital 2, 34, 35, 56
St Thomas Street 2, 3
St Thomas Street blue plaque 3, 50
St Thomas Street digs 3, 36, 37, 49, 50
St Marylebone Cemetery,
  Finchley 26
Sawrey, Solomon 40
Severn, Charles 40
Severn, Emma 40
Severn, Joseph 40, 45, 57
Snow, John 16, 19
Society of Apothecaries 2, 48
Somers, Benjamin 1
Sonnet to the Stars 7, 8,
South, John Flint 4, 28, 46, 51
Southwark 10, 11, 35, 49
Stamford Street 11, 21

Stephens
Anne, née Reilly (1814-95) 19, 27
Catherine (1763-1843) 1, 10
Catherine (b.1846) 25
Ellen (b.1853) 25, 27
Frances (1798-1860) 1
Hannah, née Woodbridge (1804-32)
  .... 12, 16, 45
Harold (b.1848) 25
Harriot (1830-31) 12, 16
Henry (1796-1864) 1, 7, 8, 15,
  17, 22, 25, death 26,28,31,36,49,56,60
Henry Charles (1841-1918)
  .. 6, 20, 25, 26, death 27, marriage 55, 56
Jennifer (b.1931) 11, 28
John (1795-1846) 55
Joseph (1771-1820) 1, 10
Julian (b.1855) 25, 27
Margaret Agnes, née Mackereth
  (b.1841) 26, 53, 54, 55
Martha (1843-1927) 17, 20, 25, 55
Samuel Josiah (1804-65)
  ....1, 12, 19, 25, 26, 55
The Stephens Collection 25, 56
Swan and Hoop 31, 32

T

Treaty of Versailles 23
Trinity College, Cambridge 36
Tuberculosis 11, 12, 33, 40, 41, 44, 45
Tyrrell, Frederick 36
Tyrrell, John 3

U

University College School,
  Hampstead 25, 55

V

Venereal disease 40

W

Walsh, Martha, née Stephens
  (b.1843) 6, 17, 20, 25, 28, 55
Watling Street 1
Well Walk, Hampstead 40, 41
Wellcome Library 13, 19
Weston Underwood, Bucks 11
Winkfield, John 1, 2, 9
Woodbridge, Hannah (1804-32)
  .... 12, 16, 45
Wordsworth, William 38, 39